T0199887

PHYSICIAN
SEXUAL
MISCONDUCT

PHYSICIAN
SEXUAL
MISCONDUCT

Edited by

Joseph D. Bloom, M.D.

Carol C. Nadelson, M.D.

Malkah T. Notman, M.D.

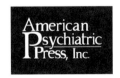

Washington, DC
London, England

Note: The authors have worked to ensure that all information in this book concerning drug dosages, schedules, and routes of administration is accurate as of the time of publication and consistent with standards set by the U.S. Food and Drug Administration and the general medical community. As medical research and practice advance, however, therapeutic standards may change. For this reason and because human and mechanical errors sometimes occur, we recommend that readers follow the advice of a physician who is directly involved in their care or the care of a member of their family.

Copyright © 1999 American Psychiatric Press, Inc.
ALL RIGHTS RESERVED
Manufactured in the United States of America on acid-free paper
02   01   00   99   4   3   2
First Edition

American Psychiatric Press, Inc.
1400 K Street, N.W., Washington, DC   20005
www.appi.org

Library of Congress Cataloging-in-Publication Data
Physician sexual misconduct / edited by Joseph D. Bloom, Carol C.
    Nadelson, Malkah T. Notman. — 1st ed.
         p.   cm.
    Includes bibliographical references and index.
    ISBN 0-88048-706-2
    1. Physician and patient—Moral and ethical aspects.
    2. Physicians—Sexual behavior—Moral and ethical aspects.
    3. Sexually abused patients—Rehabilitation.   4. Sex crimes—
    Prevention.   5. Sex between psychotherapist and patient—Moral and
    ethical aspects.—6. Physicians—Professional ethics—Study and
    teaching.   I. Bloom, Joseph D.   II. Notman, Malkah T.
    [DNLM: 1. Physician-Patient Relations.   2. Sexual Harassment.
    3. Sex Offenses—prevention & control.   4. Ethics, Medical.
    5. Malpractice.   6. Liability, Legal.   W 62S5182   1999]
    R727.3.S4745   1999
    174′.2—dc21
    DNLM/DLC
    for Library of Congress   98-27810
                                                                                        CIP

British Library Cataloguing in Publication Data
A CIP record is available from the British Library.

CONTENTS

SECTION I

Forensic Issues

CONTRIBUTORS

Gene G. Abel, M.D.
Director, Behavioral Medicine Institute of Atlanta, Atlanta, Georgia

Elissa P. Benedek, M.D.
Clinical Professor of Psychiatry, University of Michigan Medical Center, Ann Arbor, Michigan

Joseph D. Bloom, M.D.
Dean, School of Medicine, Professor of Psychiatry, Oregon Health Sciences University, Portland, Oregon

Glen O. Gabbard, M.D.
Bessie Walker Callaway Distinguished Professor of Psychoanalysis and Education, Karl Menninger School of Psychiatry and Mental Health Sciences, The Menninger Clinic; Training and Supervising Analyst, Topeka Institute for Psychoanalysis; Clinical Professor of Psychiatry, University of Kansas School of Medicine, Topeka, Kansas

Thomas G. Gutheil, M.D.
Professor of Psychiatry, Harvard Medical School; Co-Director of the Program in Psychiatry and the Law, Massachusetts Mental Health Center, Boston, Massachusetts

Jerald Kay, M.D.
Professor and Chair, Department of Psychiatry, Wright State University School of Medicine, Dayton, Ohio

Harvey Klevit, M.D.
Vice President, Medical Affairs, Physician's Association of Clackamas County Health Plans, Clackamas, Oregon

Duncan C. MacCourt, J.D.
Research Assistant, Harvard Law School, Cambridge, Massachusetts

Deane B. McCraith, M.S., O.T.R./L., L.M.F.T.
Clinical Associate Professor, Boston University—Sargent College of Allied Health Professionals, Boston, Massachusetts

Carol C. Nadelson, M.D.
Clinical Professor of Psychiatry, Harvard Medical School; Director, Partners Office for Women's Careers at Brigham and Women's Hospital, Boston, Massachusetts; President, CEO, and Editor-in-Chief, American Psychiatric Press, Inc., Washington, D.C.

Malkah T. Notman, M.D.
Clinical Professor of Psychiatry, Harvard Medical School, Cambridge Hospital, Cambridge, Massachusetts; Chair, Committee on Physician Health and Impairment, American Psychiatric Association, Washington, D.C.

Candice A. Osborn, M.A.
Director of Sex Offender Treatment Programs, Behavioral Medicine Institute of Atlanta, Atlanta, Georgia

Gail Erlick Robinson, M.D., F.R.C.P.C.
Professor of Psychiatry and Obstetrics/Gynecology, Co-Head, Women's Mental Health Program, Department of Psychiatry, University of Toronto and The Toronto Hospital, Toronto, Ontario, Canada

Brenda Roman, M.D.
Assistant Professor and Director of Medical Student and Mental Health Services, Department of Psychiatry, Wright State University School of Medicine, Dayton, Ohio

Alan A. Stone, M.D.
Touroff-Glueck Professor of Law and Psychiatry, Harvard Law and Medical Schools, Cambridge, Massachusetts

Larry H. Strasburger, M.D.
Assistant Clinical Professor of Psychiatry, Harvard Medical School, Boston, Massachusetts

Dolores R. Thomas, M.S.W., L.I.C.S.W.
Private practice, Brookline, Massachusetts

John J. Ulwelling, M.A.
Director, The Foundation for Medical Excellence, Portland, Oregon

David Wahl, M.D.
Associate Clinical Professor of Psychiatry, University of Colorado Health Sciences Center, Denver; private practice, Lakewood, Colorado; Chair, Ethics Committee, American Psychiatric Association, Washington, D.C.

Mary H. Williams, M.S., J.D.
Assistant Attorney General, State of Oregon; Adjunct Assistant Professor, Department of Psychiatry, Oregon Health Sciences University, Portland, Oregon

Janet W. Wohlberg, M.S., A.B.D.
President, The Rappay Group; Founder, TELL (Therapy Exploitation Link Line), Williamstown, Massachusetts

FOREWORD
Defining the Issues

Malkah T. Notman, M.D., Carol C. Nadelson, M.D., and Joseph D. Bloom, M.D.

This book grew out of years of work with physicians who had sexually abused patients, and with abused patients. The work took place in many contexts: treatment situations, impaired physician committees, licensing boards, ethics committees, and forensic assessments. Until recently, sexual misconduct was not openly discussed within the medical profession or publicly. Patients who complained were often accused of distorting the facts, of being in some way responsible for what had happened, or of lying. Most physicians have known colleagues who became sexually involved with current or former patients, but our profession frequently discounted the seriousness of the problem. Even when the information appeared unequivocal, there were few clear pathways for action.

This situation has changed. Sexual misconduct by physicians now receives extensive coverage and commentary in both the popular press and professional circles. There is greater awareness of this problem in the professional literature, while licensing boards and ethics committees of professional societies have taken more direct action when they receive complaints of sexual misconduct (Gabbard 1989; Schoener et al. 1989).

This book focuses on some controversial aspects of physician sexual misconduct. It concentrates on legal and ethical issues, but it also examines therapeutic and rehabilitative approaches to sexual misconduct because there is a considerable variety of opinions about whether, when, and how rehabilitation of physicians who have been involved in sexual misconduct can occur.

Greater attention to the problem of sexual misconduct on the part of professionals must also be understood in the context of a number of significant social changes. There is increased public attention to acts of sexual aggression such as rape and incest, and increased discussion of victims' rights. The women's movement has focused attention on the exploitation of women in a variety of circumstances and on the dynamics of male-female relationships in society. There is also extensive public and professional discussion of sexual harassment. The press has increasingly reported abuses committed by many professionals, including teachers, priests, ministers, and lawyers, as well as physicians and others with similar fiduciary responsibilities and obligations. All of these factors have contributed to a more open discussion of sexual misconduct.

Although the prohibition against sexual involvement with patients is explicitly stated in the Hippocratic Oath (Edelstein 1967) and reiterated in many codes of ethics (American Psychiatric Association 1998; Council on Ethical and Judicial Affairs 1991), the need to actually do something in response to infractions of this prohibition did not begin to be felt until very recently. Actions began in the courts with an increasing number of civil suits against physicians, and some medical boards and professional societies began to develop procedures for the enforcement of standards. It was not until 1990 that the Council on Ethical and Judicial Affairs of the American Medical Association took the important step of condemning sexual relations with patients as unethical.

There is now a growing international interest in the problem. Although sexual misconduct in the medical profession was informally acknowledged in many other countries, it was initially viewed as predominantly a problem in the United States. This is no longer the case. Extensive reports documenting problems and proposing mechanisms for dealing with them have recently emerged from Canada (as described by Robinson in Chapter 6). These reports were sparked in part by public outrage stirred by particularly egregious cases.

In 1994, two of us (CCN, MTN) met with medical boards in Australia and New Zealand and found similar problems and concerns. The Medical Council of New Zealand (1992) issued a statement that in effect summarized the contemporary view of physician sexual misconduct. The Council asserted that

> The ethical doctor-patient relationship depends upon the doctor creating an environment where mutual respect and trust can exist and where the patient can have confidence and safety.
>
> The onus is always on the doctor to behave in a professional manner. The community must be confident that personal boundaries will be maintained and that as patients they will never be at risk. It is never acceptable to blame the patient for the sexual misconduct.
>
> The doctor is in an uniquely privileged position regarding physical and emotional proximity. Boundaries can easily be broken in this environment.
>
> Breaches of the doctor-patient relationship risk causing psychological damage to the patient. Sexual misconduct by a doctor inevitably harms the patient.
>
> The doctor-patient relationship is not one of equality. In seeking assistance, guidance and treatment, the patient is vulnerable. Exploitation of the patient is an abuse of power. Because of the power imbalance patient consent can never be a defense.
>
> Sexual involvement with the patient leads to impairment of clinical judgement.

This powerful statement captures the current consensus about the impropriety of sexual relations between physician and patient. However, although we are clearer in some areas, we continue to struggle in other areas where continuing controversy, uncertainty, or ambiguity exists. These involve, for example, judgments as to when a doctor-patient relationship is actually established; how long it exists; and when it has ended. Are there differences in expectations between patient and doctor when there are brief professional relationships, such as a consultation, as opposed to longer-term relationships, such as those which occur between physician and patient in psychotherapy or in a primary care practice? Other gray areas include concerns about the nature of transference in medical as well as mental health settings, the patient's ability to give consent, the patient's autonomy or right to choose, and the definition of boundary violations. There are also less esoteric but nevertheless pertinent competing interests such as those between insurers, victims, and abusers. Insurers do not want to insure physicians against sexual misconduct because of the financial risk; victims have an interest in being compensated, which is not likely to occur if the physician is not insured; and physicians have less personal financial risk if they are insured. There is also controversy about whether sexual misconduct should be criminalized, and, finally, there is controversy about the treatment and rehabilitation of physicians who are determined to be guilty of sexual misconduct.

This book was designed to explore specific issues within the broad topic of sexual misconduct. It includes the perspectives of professional organizations, medical boards, forensic experts, the insurance industry, and patients. Interwoven in the book is material that pertains to physicians and/or to psychotherapists, a group that includes a wide variety of mental health professionals. The focus on both physicians and psychotherapists may at times be confusing to the reader. However, it reflects the state of current debate about the intersection of roles and ethical obligations.

In addressing the problem of sexual misconduct of physicians there may also appear to be disproportionate attention to psychiatrists and other nonphysician therapists. This occurs because there has been more attention in the literature to psychiatrists and other mental health professions. Much of what has been written, however, has direct relevance to other branches of medicine. Although the nature of the therapeutic relationship for psychiatrists may be different than for many other physicians, when a doctor-patient relationship involves long-term treatment and complex interaction, many of the same considerations apply. For example, many have discussed the difference in the transference, which is the central instrument of long-term psychotherapy, as compared with other medical treatment. However, even if it is not recognized or explicitly acknowledged, transference is a powerful factor in all physician-patient relationships, although it may be attenuated in brief encounters.

Furthermore, as the health care system changes, the distinction between physicians, psychotherapists, and other providers of health care has become more blurred. Managed care programs often encourage primary care physicians to assume more responsibility for mental health–related care. In addition, many specialties, including family medicine, pediatrics, internal medicine, and neurology are developing "behavioral" specialists who are not psychiatrists. Many states have also adopted statutory definitions of "psychotherapists" for the purpose of defining psychotherapist-patient privilege (see for example, Oregon 1993) or for use in statutes that criminalize sexual misconduct (see Chapter 2). These statutes clearly define physicians as psychotherapists, and in many of their roles physicians are clearly acting as psychotherapists for their patients.

The book is divided into four sections containing chapters on forensic issues, ethical and regulatory issues, physician education, and therapeutic and rehabilitative issues.

The section on forensic issues contains chapters on civil and criminal law related to sexual misconduct. In Chapter 1, Gutheil discusses civil litigation and the dilemmas posed by the definition of wrongdoing in malpractice cases. The relationship between the harm created and the requirements for demonstrating malpractice, as well as the insurance strategies developed by the insurance industry, complicate the picture. In this chapter Gutheil also develops a topology of abusers and of patients, a theme that Gabbard has also undertaken.

In Chapter 2, Strasburger examines the trend toward making sexual contact between psychotherapist and patient a criminal act and provides an analysis of the pros and cons of criminalization.

In Chapter 3, Stone and MacCourt address the complex issues of insurance coverage for sexual misconduct, and the dilemmas of the insurance industry and their vulnerability to loss from the large settlements of recent years. They review the history of the insurance industry's response to the problem of sexual misconduct and the competing interests of providing compensation to those harmed by such behavior.

Section II focuses on ethical and regulatory concerns related to sexual misconduct. In Chapter 4, Benedek and Wahl review the ethics, policies, and practices of the American Psychiatric Association and the American Medical Association. They set these in a clinical context, describing five examples of ethical dilemmas involving current or past physician-patient relationships.

Bloom, Williams, Ulwelling, and Klevit, in Chapter 5, discuss the role of medical boards in dealing with problems of sexual misconduct by physicians. Their data are based on both the experience of the Oregon Board of Medical Examiners and a national survey. This chapter also contains data about nonpsychiatric physicians. The authors describe differences in the way medical boards handle complaints as well as differences in outcome, including whether the physician is allowed to remain in practice. These raise questions about uniformity of approach by medical boards, as well as how well medical boards are succeeding in protecting patients and regulating medical practice.

In Chapter 6, Robinson describes the way that these issues came to public attention in Ontario in 1990 via an unusual case in which a practice called "pelvic bonding" escaped professional censure because of the narrowness of the regulatory requirements, only to create public uproar when reported by the press. Robinson traces the development of a task force on sexual abuse of patients by physicians and the effect this has had on understanding, regulation, and education in Canada.

Section III focuses on the role of education, which should be viewed as one of the most potentially effective means of prevention of sexual misconduct. Focus on the harmful effects on patients and the need for an understanding of the power of the doctor-patient relationship to the patient, as well as the acquisition of skills for dealing with the physician's own feelings are requisite components of an educational program. In Chapter 7, Kay and Roman discuss educational goals and methods, review the literature, and offer a possible course outline for a 4-year program to teach ethics to medical students. They also stress the importance of a longitudinal approach and the conditions that make for success.

Although one reason given by those proposing criminal sanctions is the failure of educational efforts to rectify the problem, educational programs at all levels have not been in place for very long, nor have there been sustained efforts to develop them. How effective these are and how educable physicians will be must be assessed over time.

Therapeutic and rehabilitative considerations are addressed in the last, and perhaps the most controversial, section of the book. Wohlberg, McCraith, and Thomas present the perspective of the survivor in Chapter 8. They review the dynamics of abuse, describe a typology of both abuser and victim, and refocus the issues, describing the process of healing and recovery for the victim. From their perspective, few perpetrators can be rehabilitated.

This view is not entirely shared by Gabbard (Chapter 9), nor by Abel and Osborn (Chapter 10), who describe primarily rehabilitative and therapeutic approaches to sexual misconduct. Gabbard discusses psychodynamic therapeutic approaches, the conditions for effective psychotherapy, and some of the countertransference dilemmas. Abel and Osborn, who have an extensive background in the evaluation and treatment of sexual abusers in the general population, outline techniques for cognitive-behavioral treatment.

Because there is a range of pathology and dynamics characterizing individuals who are abusers, success of rehabilitative and therapeutic efforts will vary with the particular population considered. As Gutheil indicates in Chapter 1, the question of whether sexual misconduct occurs because the abuser has a mental disorder is not always easily determined. Although the particular typologies proposed vary somewhat, there are also physicians who have serious character defects or are "bad actors," rather than having treatable psychiatric disorders. They may be exploitative and opportunistic toward patients, with little ability to perceive their patients' needs or feelings, and may even believe that they have done nothing wrong. Psychotherapy is unlikely to be helpful to these individuals. Perhaps the approaches outlined by Abel and Osborn in their chapter might be more effective with such individuals. However, more experience is necessary and more data must be accumulated about effective treatment and rehabilitative approaches, which will ultimately lead to a better understanding of those who would benefit from treatment and those who cannot be rehabilitated.

Successful programs have been developed for physicians with substance abuse and from psychiatric disorders, often in conjunction with medical societies and licensing boards. In 1973 the American Medical Association (Council on Mental Health 1973) focused attention on the development of programs for "impaired physicians"—those with substance abuse and mental illness. There has been significant progress in this area, although there are geographic variations (Shore 1987; Talbott et al. 1987). These programs rely on consultation (Bloom et al. 1991), treatment, and monitoring and are backed by threatened or actual suspension of the medical license. Even when a physician's behavior does not come to the attention of the board initially, if the referral comes from some other source, the possibility of reporting exists if the physician does not comply with the proscribed treatment and monitoring agreements.

Similar rehabilitative program development has not occurred in cases of sexual misconduct. Some medical societies have attempted to include sexual misconduct under the umbrella of impairment, but there are often disagreements about whether this behavior occurred because of impairment or whether it should be treated as an ethical violation or malpractice. There is also no monitoring approach for sexual misconduct that is equivalent to urine or blood screening for drugs and alcohol. Mandating a chaperone or forbidding solo practice may certainly reduce risk in many situations, such as in family medicine or obstetrics/gynecology. It is not, however, a solution for those who work with patients in psychotherapy or family counseling where individual one-to-one treatment occurs and confidentiality is critical to that treatment. In such situations chaperones are not workable.

The larger subject of boundary violations (Gabbard and Nadelson 1995; Gutheil and Gabbard 1993) provides a context for teaching about sexual misconduct. These areas are also emphasized by Notman and Nadelson in Chapter 11. They focus on psychotherapy with patients previously abused by other therapists.

All physicians, not only psychiatrists, should be better able to recognize the emotional needs of their patients. They also should be more self-aware and recognize their own potential vulnerability when they encounter career and life cycle changes and other stresses—such as losses, separations, and heightened work stress—which can increase their susceptibility to many kinds of problems, including sexual misconduct. Physicians should recognize the need for nonpunitive consultation and supervision whether they are in practice or in training. Informal discussion can be more effective than lectures.

Finally, all physicians must take responsibility for improving the current situation, for the development of training programs, and for greater public awareness of the problem of sexual misconduct. They must work within professional societies, where possible, to diminish denial and discomfort in dealing with these issues. Medical boards, through their authority and power over a physician's ability to practice, have an effective means to exert control over sexual misconduct. Some licensing boards are inexperienced with these problems and appear to alternate between polarized attitudes of permissiveness and punitiveness. This may occur because boards vary in composition and function from state to state as well as from time to time. They need to be educated to be consistent and fair.

It is our hope that the this book will further the productive discussion of physician sexual misconduct and contribute to a process of change and the development of enlightened and effective practices.

References

American Psychiatric Association: The Principles of Medical Ethics With Annotations Especially Applicable to Psychiatry. Washington, DC, American Psychiatric Association, 1998

Bloom JD, Resnick M, Ulwelling JJ, et al: Psychiatric consultation to a state board of medical examiners. Am J Psychiatry 148:1366–1370, 1991

Council on Ethical and Judicial Affairs, American Medical Association: Sexual misconduct in the practice of medicine. JAMA 266:2741–2745, 1991

Council on Mental Health: The sick physician: impairment by psychiatric disorders, including alcoholism and drug dependence. JAMA 223:684–687, 1973

Edelstein L: Ancient Medicine. Baltimore, MD, Johns Hopkins University Press, 1967

Gabbard GO (ed): Sexual Exploitation in Professional Relationships. Washington, DC, American Psychiatric Press, 1989

Gabbard GO, Nadelson C: Professional boundaries in the physician-patient relationship. JAMA 273:1445–1449, 1995

Gutheil TG, Gabbard GO: The concept of boundaries in clinical practice: theoretical and risk-management dimensions. Am J Psychiatry 150:188–196, 1993

Medical Council of New Zealand: Sexual abuse in the doctor-patient relationship. Bulletin of the Medical College of New Zealand 6:4–5, 1992

Oregon: Oregon Revised Statutes 40.230, 1993

Schoener GR, Milgrom JH, Gonsiorek JC, et al: Psychotherapists' Sexual Involvement With Clients: Interventions and Prevention. Minneapolis, MN, Walk-In Counseling Center, 1989

Shore JH: The Oregon experience with impaired physicians on probation—an eight-year follow-up. JAMA 257:2931–2934, 1987

Talbott GD, Gallegos KV, Wilson PO, Porter TL: The Medical Association of Georgia's Impaired Physician Program—review of the first 1000 physicians: analysis of specialty. JAMA 257:2927–2930, 1987

SECTION I
Forensic Issues

1

ISSUES IN
CIVIL SEXUAL MISCONDUCT
LITIGATION

Thomas G. Gutheil, M.D.

S exual misconduct is a tragically widespread offense bringing distress to victims, embarrassment to the professions, dismay to insurers, glee to the media, and frustration to those interested in combating this serious modern problem (Appelbaum and Gutheil 1991; Edelwich and Brodsky 1991; Gabbard 1989; Pope and Bouhoutsos 1986; Pope et al. 1993; Rutter 1989; Schoener et al. 1989; Siegel 1991; Strean 1993). Proscribed by the ethical codes of all mental health professional organizations, sexual misconduct is increasingly in the professional and public news, though at least a part of its apparent spread may represent a "shakeout" phase, wherein media reports bring other old cases out of

I am indebted to members of the Program in Psychiatry and the Law, Massachusetts Mental Health Center, Boston, Massachusetts, for conceptual contributions, and especially to Larry Strasburger, M.D., for critical review and comments.

the closets, and hesitant victims, long silent, decide to risk the stresses of public accusation of abusers. Estimates of the prevalence of this harm suffer the beclouding effects of underreporting, methodological problems with questionnaire studies, the power of rumor, political overestimation, and similar forces. Scholars of the harm it can do come to feel that "any is too many," but effective prevention remains a persisting conundrum.

Careful study of the problem almost immediately stumbles on the rock of political correctness: in some circles discussion of this issue is heresy if it proceeds in any terms *other* than that of a true story of a psychopathic, predatory therapist and passive victim. There are several reasons for embracing this model (Gutheil and Gabbard 1992). First, it appeals to one's sense of simplicity; second, it appears to present victims in a sympathetic light, respecting the harms done by the abuse; third, it adheres to gender and power stereotypes; fourth, it entirely avoids blaming or even seeming to blame the victim; finally, it is an accurate picture in a number of cases—but not in all, and there is the rub. I have been publicly chastised for even mentioning in public the possibility that false claims exist, lest this further shake the credibility of victims and increase their difficulty in coming forward.

I have found it useful to begin such discussions with three axioms intended to provide a moral compass for navigating these murky waters.

Axiom I: Only the professional has a professional code to violate; the patient has no such code. Hence, only the professional can be—depending on the context—blameworthy, culpable, liable, or guilty of criminal conduct. The patient-victim *cannot* be similarly blamed.

Axiom II: In the usual (but not universal) pairing of competent adults, however, both parties may be held accountable for their actions, albeit subject to influence, fraudulent misrepresentation, passion, venality, and the like. This view, however, *cannot* either blame the victim or exonerate the professional (see Axiom I).

Axiom III: An understanding of this serious problem requires rigorous and clear-eyed empirical study, free from political "shoulds"— study that will benefit all the parties concerned by leading to preventive strategies for practitioners, patients, and professions and to eradication of this blot on our field.

Discussion of this issue draws upon my experience as expert witness and case consultant in 216 cases from (literally) Maine to California, involving all mental health disciplines, no matter how peripheral; nonpsychiatric physicians of a half-dozen specialties; clergy; and, so far, one attorney. The intrinsic complexity of this group of cases is augmented by the fact that a small number of the cases are probably false claims (although most are probably true); some involve erotized boundary violations (Gutheil and Gabbard 1993; Simon 1991, 1992; Simon and Epstein 1990) without actual intercourse; and a small number overlap with the issue of "recovered memory," itself a subject of great complexity (Gutheil 1993).

The Context of Civil Litigation

Unlike criminal law, which deals primarily with violation of laws (statutes), civil litigation deals with disputes between people; tort law is the segment of civil law that concerns civil wrongs leading to losses. Professional malpractice is one such tort, or civil wrong.

The essence of malpractice may be summarized mnemonically by the "four Ds" of malpractice litigation: *dereliction* of a *duty directly* causing *damages*. Each of these elements requires explication in relation to sexual misconduct.

Clinicians who assume the care of a patient owe that patient a *duty* of reasonable care in assessment and treatment. In a malpractice case the patient (now called the plaintiff) claims that the defendant doctor was derelict in this duty, in that the doctor allegedly deviated from the "standard of [reasonable] care." The standard of care is a theoretical level of quality of practice usually expressed (in case law or statute) in such language as "the care of the average reasonable practitioner"; "the care of the average prudent practitioner"; or "the care rendered by a practitioner at the same level of training and specialization."

A practitioner who has sex with a patient is clearly deviating from contemporary standards of psychiatric practice. But mere deviation does not constitute malpractice. The plaintiff must also prove in court that this deviation *directly* caused physical, emotional, or economic damages (sometimes described as harms or losses). For example, a patient who has had sexual relations with a therapist might suffer, as a direct result, from depression, anxiety, and distrust of future treaters;

these symptoms would represent the emotional harms of the case. The "cost" of these damages—the dollar value ultimately assigned to these losses by the jury—would constitute the "award" as compensation for the alleged malpractice.

This already complex process is further complicated by considerations of attorneys' legal strategy and some principles of reimbursement by malpractice insurers, as described below.

The Attorney's Ploy, the Insurer's Dilemma

Some of the earliest cases in sexual misconduct civil litigation (e.g., *Roy v. Hartogs*) encountered the problem that remains to the present: what insurance posture is the most appropriate to the situation and from whose viewpoint? To understand the issue fully we must analyze the problem encountered by the plaintiff's (i.e., patient's) attorney in deciding to bring a malpractice suit for sexual misconduct against a therapist. Such suits are generally considered not worth undertaking unless the litigation develops access to the therapist's malpractice insurance policy. Bringing suit in a context that leads to large available funds worth winning is referred to in the legal profession as the "deep pockets" doctrine.

As tempting a target as an insurance policy may be, its payment is reserved for suits about negligence; that is, "sins of omission," or negligent torts. Insurers held that sexual misconduct was a fully intentional wrongful act (intentional tort) and thus not covered by a malpractice insurance policy. The problem for the plaintiff's attorney could now be formulated: how can I turn an intentional tort into a negligent one (which would permit access to the malpractice insurance policy)?

The solution hit upon was to present the claim as negligence in the management of transference and countertransference. Although this model would seem to be limited in application to cases of psychoanalysis or analytically oriented psychotherapy, it has been applied to all forms of therapy, even those that eschew this conceptual model. Indeed, some courts have proved curiously susceptible to this way of thinking, even to say in essence, in *Zipkin v. Freeman* and in *St. Paul Fire and Marine v. Love,* that the sexual contact was irrelevant to the issue; it was the abuse of transference that was the wrongdoing. How these can be separated in this manner is a judicial conundrum.

Practitioners in ideological groupings that omit discussion of transference dynamics (such as behavioral or psychopharmacological psychiatry) might claim to be excluded from claims of wrongdoing for sexual misconduct. It is unmistakably clear, however, that in the present climate such a defense would be ignored: misconduct is wrong no matter what the therapeutic ideology.

Insurers who thus bear the brunt of such litigation have used several strategies to minimize risks and conserve resources. Some policies place a cap on the outlay of funds for misconduct suit defenses; others refuse all payment. Each approach presents some advantages and some disadvantages from the viewpoint of social benefits.

Insurers who pay nothing—neither funds for defense nor awards for a plaintiff's victory—act as the strongest deterrent to clinicians engaging in sexual misconduct, since all costs are borne out of pocket; however, under this model, victims may be denied compensation for future treatment and damages.

Insurers who pay for the defense but not a plaintiff's award permit some screening out of the minority of false claims but do not deter clinicians as forcibly, nor do they provide victims with compensation.

Insurers who pay both defense and loss costs provide social benefits in compensation but do not serve as a strong deterrent to errant practitioners.

Terminology

A number of terms have been employed to describe, or describe aspects of, the situation wherein a professional has sexual relations in some form with a patient or client either during treatment or so shortly afterward that it amounts to the same thing; the terms convey a range of nuances that may be important for forming conceptual models or for presenting clear testimony to a confused jury in a civil case.

Sexual misconduct locates the problem in the erotic arena and stresses the wrongness of the conduct, presumably from the ethical viewpoint. It is a relatively neutral term.

Abuse reflects abuse of the fiduciary (trust-based) relationship between professional and patient, abuse of transference and power asymmetry in some cases, and harm to the patient. However, since sexual relations with therapists can endure for years on a weekly basis (decades-long relations are encountered in practice), the expert encounters trouble in using this term before juries: they reason, if it is abuse, why did the patient seek it weekly for years? As will later be addressed, the abusive nature of the relationship may not be appreciated at first. Of course, abuse pure and simple does occur, as when a patient is drugged and raped during treatment; fortunately, this is rare.

Deviation conveys the idea of divergence from a standard of care, one of the elements of malpractice (Appelbaum and Gutheil 1991). Although the deviation is clear, insurers may locate sexual relations as entirely outside the pale of clinical practice, so that a traditional malpractice analysis does not apply and they need not pay.

Harm proves to be a frequent consequence of sexual misconduct; few patients are unscathed by it. If they are unharmed (in a minority of cases), it is usually when they take the initiative (Pope and Bouhoutsos 1986) in sexual relations.

Exploitation captures the fundamental wrongness of the relationship even if it appears to be occurring between "consenting adults": no matter how gratifying the relationship, it places the patient's needs for good therapy second to having sex or to the therapist's needs. Hence, sexual misconduct is always exploitative.

Violation often applies: both boundaries (Gutheil and Gabbard 1993; Simon 1991, 1992; Simon and Epstein 1990) and fiduciary requirements are violated, as are ethical codes. It may be noteworthy that many of my most recent cases do not involve actual intercourse but instead, highly eroticized boundary violations. Though really no less exploitative than intercourse, such boundary cases may well represent the wave of the future, as therapists—now aware of the wrongness of sex with patients—become involved in this arena instead.

Fitness to practice may be questioned in the context of a complaint to a board of registration or licensing. Recidivist psychopathic therapists best fit this model, since future offense is likely and rehabilitative efforts are largely foredoomed. Other categories of therapists, discussed below, may be rehabilitated successfully.

Trauma represents one of the more complex issues in this area. Relationships between patients and therapists can endure for prolonged periods—even decades, as noted above—often fueled by the patients' feelings of being unique (specially chosen) and by patients perceiving the relationship as a bond with someone who understands them perfectly. This shallow but gratifying perception may endure until one of two common trigger events occurs.

The first is the patient finding out, from media or rumor or other source, that the therapist is involved in this supposedly "unique" relationship with another patient. The second is the therapist disappointing the patient in some abandonment-related way: refusing to leave his wife; going on a prolonged vacation; attempting to stop, or stopping, the therapy; and the like. Such acts appear to shatter the patient's perceptions of the specialness of the situation, and the entire relationship undergoes a catastrophic reinterpretation—a *peripeteia,* in the terms of Greek tragedy—whereby the essentially exploitative nature of the relationship explosively dawns on the patient. At *that* point the patient may have a fully formed episode of posttraumatic stress disorder or related phenomena such as anxiety, depression, suicidal preoccupations, and the like, unleashed by the *cessation* of the relationship—hence my term *cessation trauma* (Gutheil 1991).

I depict the previous gratifying relationship as resembling a steadily stretching rubber band (the stretching representing the latent and underlying destructive potential in the situation) that tightens over time, then snaps at the point of the trigger event. Such metaphors may clarify for jurors and others that the seeds of the trauma were latent in the pathologic relationship from the outset, but the trauma stands revealed only at its end.

Typologies

Scholars in the field of sexual misconduct appear to have a fondness for creating typologies of abusers (Gabbard 1989; Gutheil 1989b; Irons, in press; Pope and Bouhoutsos 1986; Stone 1984), and I am no exception. The value of such taxonomy lies in the potential it offers to intervene and respond to misconduct based on individual case circumstances. My own typology overlaps quite well with others (e.g., Stone's eight types [Stone 1984], Gabbard's depiction of the "lovesick," the "psychotic," and the "psychopathic" therapist [Gabbard 1989]) and derives directly from my experience noted above.

In the case of male therapists, the first and most common category is the therapist in midlife crisis whose marriage, career, and life stage are not going well; this therapist encounters a patient whose particular chemistry appears to promise salvation, redemption, a cure for boredom, and a validation of his therapeutic skills. Later, the patient may supply reassurance of the therapist's sexual desirability as well. Simon (1989) describes the pathognomonic early response of both parties as "Where have you been all my life?" Indeed, such an initial response may well be a clinical indication of the need for referral, on the basis of a problematic preconceived countertransference.

The process of misconduct usually begins with boundary violations, often progressing from subtle to gross, and begins to include deep and personal self-disclosure; the latter trend may induce a role reversal when the therapist's confiding in the patient serves as a conscious or even unconscious bid for help, support, gratification, and, sometimes, "treatment" of the therapist by the patient. This role reversal is particularly likely to lead to sexual misconduct (G. R. Schoener, personal communication, May 1994).

Therapists in midlife crisis tend to single out one particular patient because of a chemistry peculiar to that dyad. The prognosis for treatment and rehabilitation is usually good, although recidivism and an exploitative history are poor prognostic signs.

A second category is the mentally ill therapist, usually with a psychotic disorder, usually of the affective type. Substance abuse is also fairly common in the abusing therapist. The common forms of Axis I disorder encountered are usually mania or hypomania—or, in some cases, extreme pathological narcissism rising near the threshold of mania—with accompanying hypersexuality and boundary weakness. Here, the prognosis is that of the underlying disorder. Severely narcissistic therapists are often recidivists and manifest a generally poor prognosis.

A third type encountered is the therapist with psychopathic or antisocial personality disorder. No professional school or discipline appears to be capable of weeding out such individuals by the usual screening methods. One scholar has noted (L. L. Havens, personal communication, April 1971) that the differential diagnosis of psychopathy includes normalcy because of the skill at social mimicry possessed by such individuals (extending at times to imposture). Psychopathic therapists tend to be polyexploiters; that is, they recidivistically exploit multiple patients and exploit those patients in multiple ways: sexually, financially, dependently, ethically, morally, socially, and so on. One such individual showed one patient nude photographs of another patient. In another example, a therapist contrived to have sexual relations with a female patient while she was still groggy from just having had electroconvulsive therapy. Another psychopathic therapist behaved similarly when his female patients were under the influence of amobarbital sodium.

In a notorious Massachusetts case, a psychopathic male therapist had sexual relations, and shared drugs and alcohol, in his office with several male patients. With one patient as spectator, he perpetrated an imposture, passing himself off as a famous comedian. He also persuaded an adult male patient to obtain a circumcision to improve their sexual relations. The prognosis is poor for treatment or rehabilitation, and removal from the profession and revocation of licensure appear to be the only suitable responses.

A fourth type is the schizoid or paraphilic therapist for whom the sexual misconduct, often with strong voyeuristic or exhibitionistic themes, is not even an element of a true relationship; instead, the exploitation is directed at gratification of a paraphilia. Treatment here is among the most difficult in the field, and the prognosis for success is poor.

Women therapists who sexually abuse patients fall into two major types in my experience. The first is the histrionic (what used to be called "hysteric," that is, struggling with oedipal-stage issues) therapist who becomes flooded with poorly integrated sexual feelings about a (usually male) patient and loses her grip on boundaries and professional limits. In one case in the western United States, the female counselor began commenting in the very first session with a troubled male patient, "You look kinda like a cowboy; I've always wanted to date a cowboy," and things proceeded (downhill) from there. The prognosis here for the therapist's future behavior is fairly good, in that short-term therapy and psychoeducational efforts, coupled with supervision, are usually successful.

The more common scenario—the most common female therapist paradigm—is that of the therapist of a lesbian orientation who becomes involved with a heterosexual or lesbian female patient. Such relationships—radical feminist theory about gender absolutes notwithstand-ing—can be fully as exploitative and destructive as those involving male therapists. For example, a lesbian social worker consulted me be-cause a client was threatening to sue her. Apparently, this was the third case in which a client had become a lover, usually only a few weeks into treatment; it became clear that this therapist was using her professional status as a way to find available lesbian partners.

These relationships usually begin with the therapist adopting a nur-turing and supportive role, generating an essentially maternal transfer-ence; this gradually becomes genitally erotized, and sexual relations or other boundary violations occur. Some of these relationships manifest high degrees of ego boundary compromise and fusion (Gutheil 1991). For example, one lesbian therapist would arrange to go to the office bathroom at the same time as her straight patient and contrive to take the adjoining stall while carrying on the conversation through the stall wall; later, when the relationship had become fully sexualized and the therapist was spending the night at the patient's house, the therapist would contrive to wear the patient's clothes to work the following day (Gutheil 1991).

One defendant in a lawsuit made the point that the lesbian subcul-ture is at present very restricted and often confined to a set circle of bars, clubs, etc., where the possibility of lesbian therapists encounter-ing their own lesbian patients is quite high; this essentially cultural fac-tor may predispose to the risk of boundary violations and may well challenge responsible lesbian therapists to maintain boundary limits successfully. Although they are less common empirically, relationships between gay male therapists and male patients may reveal similar subcultural influences.

The Patients

A variety of patients similarly present in cases of sexual misconduct, and some controversy arises as well (Gutheil 1989a); the reader may wish to consider again the axioms provided at the beginning of this chapter.

Vulnerability appears to be the single most common factor in pa-tients who become sexually involved with therapists. The vulnerability may stem from present distress, recent loss, dependency, a psycho-physiologic "addiction" to abusive relationships (Van der Kolk 1989), or similar forces. In a malignant complement to this vulnerability, therapists often initiate what is termed "grooming" behavior, designed both to assess the patient's likelihood of compliance and to initiate a shift from a professional to a personal relationship. One male therapist commented to his female patient, "I don't understand how you can be so unhappy when you have such a beautiful body." The patient's response, fortunately, was, "I think we need a consultation." But it appears that too many patients cannot or do not respond in this constructive way.

Borderline patients appear empirically to dominate the field of *litigants* in sexual misconduct cases (Gutheil 1989a). This finding does not imply, as some have claimed (Jordan et al. 1990), that "if misconduct, then borderline," since the pool of litigants is not necessarily congruent with the pool of victims. We might infer that patients in other diagnostic categories may not bring litigation for a comparable offense, for a variety of inhibitory reasons. It should also be recalled that litigation requires the plaintiff to be able to sustain a "grudge," as it were, for years on end; this tenacity is a borderline trait, perhaps even, under some circumstances, a strength.

There are several possible reasons for borderline domination of the litigant pool. One theory, based on the psychodynamic features of the disorder (Gutheil 1989a), suggests that factors such as rage, entitlement, boundary confusion, psychotic transference, and the like predispose these patients to involvement. Stone has suggested (A. A. Stone, personal communication, March 1988) that psychotic patients are too impaired to attract therapists and neurotic patients are too shrewd to become involved, so that the field is left to borderline patients by a kind of diagnostic default (Gutheil 1989a). Other theorists suggest that the finding is an artifact: validly guilty therapists accuse patients of having the borderline syndrome after the suit is filed in an attempt to discredit them; or after the abuse occurs patients begin to manifest traits consistent with borderline syndrome, since sexual abuse is recognized as a shaping factor (Herman et al. 1989) in that symptom picture. Lack of training in treating borderline patients may play a role in both boundary violations and, ultimately, sexual misconduct.

I have encountered a clear comorbidity pattern of three overlapping factors: sexual abuse during childhood; eating disorder, multiple per-

sonality disorder, or borderline personality disorder; and sexual involvement with therapists in adult life (Gutheil 1992b). Forces
producing this result may include the repetition compulsion (a compulsion to repeat a traumatic experience in the service of mastery) or
psychophysiologic tropisms to maintain abusive relationships (Van
der Kolk 1989)—patients addicted to their own endorphins, it is
suggested—or the response learned in childhood that only sexualized
and/or abusive relationships are familiar, real, or authentic; all these
may create the pathologic attachments seen in misconduct. The precise
causal mechanism behind this empirical finding remains obscure.

False Claims of Sexual Misconduct

Claims of sexual misconduct are usually true but, alas for both simplicity and integrity, a small number of false claims do arise to bedevil the
investigator. We must bow to the fundamental uncertainty in the liability field by referring to such claims as apparently false in contrast to the
majority that are apparently true, acknowledging that we are eyewit-
nesses to neither (Gutheil 1992a). A number of cases, also small, must
occupy the gray zone entitled "don't know," wherein the patient says
yes, the therapist says no, the therapy has appeared to be professional
and free of boundary violations, and no other evidence from anywhere
is available either way. A guide for the forensic expert consulting on
such a case is provided elsewhere (Gutheil 1992a); we here focus only
on the clinical and risk management dimensions.

False claims may be categorized empirically as lies, delusions, distortions, and coat-tailing or conspiracy.

Lies are by far the most common; a fabricated claim is almost always
intended to punish the therapist for some perceived misdeed, often
some form of abandonment or termination. Other aspects aside, a lawsuit is a form of relationship, a hostile-dependent one to be sure; but a
patient may use litigation to prolong a connection with a therapist who
has terminated, especially if the termination is unilateral; that is, the
therapist "fires" the patient. Other cases arise from disputes over bill-
ing, when the patient hits upon a way to reverse the cash flow, as it
were.

Delusions are actually rare, despite the fact that errant therapists have been known to dismiss patients' valid accusations with this label. Examples include psychotic patients who assume that their own sexual arousal means that sex has occurred and erotomaniac situations in which the patient brings a claim based on those essentially projected feelings. One famous case involved a psychotic patient assuming that a highly erotic novel she happened to read constituted a description of her relationship with the therapist (Gutheil 1992a).

The distortion category is a particularly interesting one, described by one researcher as "true but false" (J. Herman, personal communication, January 1991). In this situation the patient's claim that sex (i.e., intercourse) occurred is distorted in that actual penetration did not occur; the relationship, however, was so boundaryless and erotized that its generic sexuality gives a certain kind of truth to the claim.

Finally, two related phenomena—coat-tailing and conspiracy—account for the remainder of this pool of false claims. Coat-tailing is the litigative equivalent in malpractice of those venal individuals who, coming upon a bus accident, leap aboard and hurl themselves to the bus floor, screaming, "Whiplash!" They thus hope to profit from an accident in which they were not validly involved. A high-profile case in the news may tempt other patients of the same clinician to advance a false claim on the coat-tails of the extant one, in the hope that the two claims will prove mutually corroborative and thus make stronger cases for both parties. Conspiracy involves the same mechanism planned in advance: in addition to the profit motive, dependent individuals may be consciously or unconsciously competing for specialness in relation to the therapist (Gutheil 1992a).

What defense can one offer against someone who is willing to lie under oath? No direct defenses, perhaps; but three indirect preventive defenses may prove effective; I have referred to these as "context" defenses (Gutheil 1992a): First, professionalism in all areas, which makes the accusation inherently implausible. Second, avoidance of any form of boundary violations (Gutheil and Gabbard 1992; Simon 1991, 1992). Third, avoidance of any forms of sexual harassment anywhere. Those who are uncertain how a workplace issue (harassment) relates to a matter of the standard of clinical practice (misconduct) may consider how a history of harassment (or, indeed, even a harassment charge) may be used to impugn the defendant's credibility around boundary issues or, if the sexes are appropriate, around women.

Conclusion

In this chapter I have attempted to draw on empirical experience in forensic consultation to outline some of the clinical and medicolegal issues involved in one of our profession's serious current problems.
Beside the "twin pillars" of liability prevention: documentation and
consultation—both applicable here—we add care in practice and in
maintaining boundaries as the essentials of risk management for the
practitioner.

References

Appelbaum PS, Gutheil TG: Clinical Handbook of Psychiatry and the Law,
    2nd Edition. Baltimore, MD, Williams & Wilkins, 1991
Edelwich J, Brodsky A: Sexual Dilemmas for the Helping Professional, 2nd
    Edition. New York, Brunner/Mazel, 1991
Gabbard GO (ed): Sexual Exploitation in Professional Relationships. Wash-
    ington, DC, American Psychiatric Press, 1989
Gutheil TG: Borderline personality disorder, boundary violations and patient-
    therapist sex. Am J Psychiatry 146:597–602, 1989a
Gutheil TG: Patient-therapist sexual relations. Harvard Medical School Men-
    tal Health Letter 6:4–6, 1989b
Gutheil TG: Patients involved in sexual misconduct with therapists: is a vic-
    tim profile possible? Psychiatric Annals 21:661–667, 1991
Gutheil TG: Approaches to forensic assessment of false allegations of sexual
    misconduct by therapists. Bulletin of the American Academy of Psychia-
    try and the Law 20:289–296, 1992a
Gutheil TG: "Therapist-patient sex syndrome": the perils of nomenclature for
    the forensic psychiatrist. Bulletin of the American Academy of Psychiatry
    and the Law 20:185–190, 1992b
Gutheil TG: True or false memories of sexual abuse? a forensic psychiatric
    view. Psychiatric Annals 23:527–531, 1993
Gutheil TG, Gabbard GO: Obstacles to the dynamic understanding of patient-
    therapist sexual relations. Am J Psychother 46:515–525, 1992
Gutheil TG, Gabbard GO: The concept of boundaries in clinical practice: the-
    oretical and risk management dimensions. Am J Psychiatry 150:188–196,
    1993

Herman JL, Perry JC, Van der Kolk BA: Childhood trauma in borderline personality disorders. Am J Psychiatry 146:490–495, 1989

Irons R: The sexually exploitative professional: an archetypal classification, in Medicine 2000. Washington, DC, American Psychiatric Press (in press)

Jordan JV, Kaplan A, Miller JB, et al: More on therapist-patient sex (letter). Am J Psychiatry 147:129–130, 1990

Pope KS, Bouhoutsos JC: Sexual Intimacy Between Therapists and Patients. New York, Praeger, 1986

Pope KS, Sonne JL, Holroyd J: Sexual Feelings in Psychotherapy. Washington, DC, American Psychological Association, 1993

Roy v Hartogs, 85 Misc 2d 891, 381 NYS2d 587 (NYAppTerm 1976)

Rutter P: Sex in the Forbidden Zone. Los Angeles, CA, Tarcher, 1989

Schoener GR, Milgrom JH, Gonsiorek JC, et al: Psychotherapists' Sexual Involvement with Clients: Intervention and Prevention. Minneapolis, MN, Walk-in Counseling Center, 1989

Siegel SJ: What to Do When Psychotherapy Goes Wrong. Seattle, WA, Stop Abuse by Counselors Publishing, 1991

Simon RI: Sexual exploitation of patients: how it begins before it happens. Psychiatric Annals 19:104–112, 1989

Simon RI: Psychological injury caused by boundary violation precursors to therapist-patient sex. Psychiatric Annals 21:614–619, 1991

Simon RI: Treatment boundary violations: clinical, ethical and legal considerations. Bulletin of the American Academy of Psychiatry and the Law 20:269–288, 1992

Simon RI, Epstein RS: The exploitation index: an early warning indicator of boundary violations in psychotherapy. Bull Menninger Clin 54:450–465, 1990

St. Paul Fire and Marine v Love, 447 NW2d 5 (Minn Ct App 1989)

Stone AA: Law, Psychiatry and Morality. Washington, DC, American Psychiatric Press, 1984, pp 191–216

Strean HS: Therapists Who Have Sex With Their Patients: Treatment and Recovery. New York, Brunner/Mazel, 1993

Stricker G, Fisher M (eds): Self Disclosure in the Therapeutic Relationship. New York, Plenum, 1990

Van der Kolk BA: The compulsion to repeat the trauma: reenactment, revictimization, and masochism. Psychiatr Clin North Am 12:389–411, 1989

Zipkin v Freeman, 436 SW2d at 761

2

"THERE OUGHTA BE A LAW"
Criminalization of Psychotherapist-Patient Sex as a Social Policy Dilemma

Larry H. Strasburger, M.D.

Awakened by banner headlines in the media, public awareness of sexual exploitation of patients by psychotherapists has been steadily increasing (Bouhoutsos et al. 1983). Julie Roy brought the matter to national attention when she filed a civil lawsuit against her psychiatrist, Renatus Hartogs, in 1975 (*Roy v. Hartogs*). The issue has continued to command front-page stories detailing the accusations of other patients who have had the courage to go public. In an episode of *Frontline,* the Public Broadcasting System televised interviews with a sexually exploited patient and her psychiatrist (Storring and Zaritsky 1991). Today, offending professionals continue to make headlines in cases all

I wish to thank Carol Strasburger and Linda Jorgenson for their kind support and assistance in the preparation of this chapter.

across the country (Epstein 1994; Gabbard 1989; Pope 1989, 1994; Pope and Bouhoutsos 1986).

Traditionally, the modes for dealing with the problem of sexual abuse of psychotherapy patients have been professional association disciplinary proceedings, civil lawsuits, and complaints to state licensing boards. Critics of the status quo, however, assert that these sanctions are not adequate to deal with the problem because they do not penalize the offending behavior sufficiently to satisfy the victims and because they do not provide adequate deterrence to continuing offenders or to others who might be contemplating misbehavior. Ethics procedures are often slow to get under way because ethics committees lack the resources (and sometimes the courage) to pursue violations of the ethical canon. Ethics committees, usually composed of volunteers, have been hampered by lack of time, lack of money to obtain adequate legal advice, and the hesitant approach of professionals uncomfortable with the issues and anxious not to be sued by the practitioners being investigated. Even the perception of this reticence to proceed undermines deterrence and increases public outrage.

A second avenue of redress, a civil malpractice lawsuit, provides money damages to a plaintiff who can prove that she or he was damaged by the negligent actions of a psychiatrist who, through sexual contact, failed in his or her professional duty. Other lawsuits have charged battery and negligent or intentional infliction of emotional distress. Such suits are costly to all concerned. A patient's ability to initiate such proceedings generally depends on finding an attorney willing to undertake the suit on a contingent fee basis. The civil courts work slowly, and it is not unusual for years to pass before they reach a judgment, which then can be appealed. A further complaint about the civil litigation process is that ultimately it is an insurance company, rather than the offending professional, that usually pays the bill. This provides little redress for victims of therapists without assets, little discouragement for the guilty therapist who may repeat the offense (though the practitioner may be dropped by the insurer), and little deterrence for other therapists. The statute of limitations may make a suit impossible when years have passed before the victim realizes the harm by making a connection between symptoms suffered and the sexual misconduct of the therapist. Indeed, the very nature of the damage caused by the abuse may prevent victims from asserting their legal rights within the statute of limitations (*Riley v. Presnell*).

Complaints to licensing boards may result in administrative prosecution, which can result in fines as well as the suspension or revocation of the practitioner's license. The psychiatrist may be required to undergo rehabilitation in the form of personal treatment and/or special education, as well as supervision or monitoring of his or her practice. There is greater flexibility to these prosecutions because the statute of limitations does not apply to licensing boards and the rules of evidence are considerably more relaxed than in court proceedings.

A shortcoming of licensing board sanctions is that the primary goal of incapacitating the offender after the suspension or revocation of license still may not be attained. "When the Massachusetts medical board started revoking the licenses of psychiatrists charged with sexual misconduct, its officials assumed their rulings would put these doctors out of business. They assumed wrong. . . . Doctors who lose their licenses are no longer allowed to prescribe medication, admit patients to hospitals or treat medical conditions, but there is no law in this state that says they can't treat patients in psychotherapy" (Bass 1993).

Most states have not regulated the practice of psychotherapy by unlicensed therapists. As an unlicensed practitioner, an offender is able to continue to misuse the therapy relationship and repeat predatory behavior. Clearly, each of the traditional remedies contains deficiencies.

Criminalization

Despite their inadequacies, powerful disincentives for professional misconduct do exist, yet a common public perception suggests that "nothing is being done" and fuels a demand for new and more substantial penalties. Is criminalization a solution (Strasburger et al. 1991)? Much of the public and many members of the professional world believe that it is. As of 1998, 16 states had passed legislation making sexual contact between psychotherapist and patient a criminal act (Arizona, California, Colorado, Connecticut, Florida, Georgia, Iowa, Maine, Minnesota, New Hampshire, New Mexico, North Dakota, South Dakota, Texas, Utah, Wisconsin).

Masters and Johnson first called for criminalization in 1975. Outraged by sexual exploitation of patients by psychotherapists, they appealed for criminalization of the behavior. "We feel that when sexual seduction of patients can be firmly established by due legal process, regardless of whether the seduction was initiated by the patient or the therapist, the therapist should initially be sued for rape rather than malpractice, i.e., the legal process should be criminal rather than civil" (Masters and Johnson 1976). Although it was controversial at the time, other clinicians, victim groups, and the public at large have amplified the recommendation.

Criminal law depends on retribution and utilitarian theories for its justification (Barker 1990, p. 1294). Retribution is basically social revenge, which is a derivative of private, personal vengeance. Retribution, then, is a morally justified retaliation. In a proportional way, retribution seeks to enact the quantity of harm on the wrongdoer that was inflicted on society, rectifying an imbalance. Suffering is meted out by a vindictive justice that pays back the wrongdoer, who receives punishment that he justly deserves because he has done wrong and inflicted harm. Retribution expresses society's moral condemnation through a concrete act of denunciation: an eye for an eye, a tooth for a tooth.

Utilitarian theory seeks deterrence—both specific deterrence by incapacitating the offender and intimidating him from repeating his offense, and general deterrence through public notice of the risks of prohibited activities. The theory assumes that by performing a risk-benefit analysis, a potential offender will learn that any pleasure or profit from misconduct will be offset by the risk of pain, inducing different choices and alternative conduct. Furthermore, it assumes that minimizing the occurrence rate of offenses provides a net benefit to society, which justifies punishment. The presence of this net benefit is crucial to the concept. Because punishment is an infliction of harm, in itself evil, it must be justified by a proportional reduction of harm to society. The utilitarian, therefore, seeks a balancing of interests: Does the prohibited behavior create a significant social harm? Does criminalizing lead to consequences that outweigh the benefits? Might means other than criminal law prevent the harm equally effectively?

An important aspect of criminalization is its due process requirements. For the psychiatrist who must defend against an accusation of sexual exploitation, the criminal justice system offers a much greater degree of protection than the procedures of either civil suits or licensing board hearings. Since the stakes are so much greater when there is a potential loss of liberty, a conviction under the criminal law requires that the jury find that the evidence indicates guilt "beyond a reasonable doubt." This standard of proof is a much higher hurdle than the civil law standard of proof by "a preponderance of the evidence," usually interpreted as simply more likely than not. Many cases involve little more in the way of evidence than allegations of misconduct in an office in which the only two persons who could have witnessed the behavior disagree with one another. The high standard of proof required for criminal prosecution will give pause to a prosecutor who might have any ambivalence about going forward with a doubtful case. Due process protection in the criminal law also provides stricter safeguards for the accused than the protection available at a licensing board hearing. Licensing boards may allow testimony that would be excluded under criminal rules of evidence, and licensing boards are not bound by a statute of limitations.

Clearly, there is a compelling state interest in protecting the health and safety of its citizens, and therapist-patient sex has been shown to be unquestionably harmful. Public debate is ongoing about whether other means of dealing with the harm are equally effective and whether the disadvantages of criminalization outweigh the benefits.

Arguments for Criminalization

Failure of the System

Supporters of criminalization cite the prevalence of psychotherapist sexual exploitation to show that the system is not working adequately to protect patients. Professional association ethics committees provide, many say, only a slap on the wrist; licensure boards are often unresponsive or impotent; civil lawsuits are an uncertain source of redress and of little value as a deterrent. None of these three social controls deals with the psychotherapist who continues to practice without a license.

Deterrence

Deterrence is the primary argument in favor of criminalization. The harm to the public is clearly articulated, and the profession is put on notice that misbehavior carries substantial risks. No insurer will stand between the offending psychiatrist and the judgment of a criminal court. Although the effectiveness of this deterrence has not been empirically demonstrated, it seems clear that a felony conviction and a prison sentence are penalties no rational psychiatrist would choose to risk. Predatory, psychotic, or impulsive psychotherapists, or those who consider themselves above the law, may not respond to potential sanctions; alternatively, exploitative psychotherapists who are naive, poorly informed, or undergoing some form of personal life crisis are likely to respond to the threat of punishment.

Retribution

Now that a substantial body of evidence exists showing the harm done to patients through sexual exploitation, it can be argued that such exploitation is so outrageous a transgression of societal rules that retribution is called for. Even if therapist misbehavior rooted in the character pathology of impulsive, narcissistic, or sociopathic personalities were not deterred by criminalization, retribution for the harm caused by these individuals would still be appropriate.

Unlicensed Therapists

Criminalization offers one means to deal with therapists who continue to practice unregulated after the licensing board revokes their licenses. Although licensing boards cannot administratively sanction these individuals, and many boards have too few resources to make a civil lawsuit worthwhile, offending therapists can be incapacitated through criminal law. While imprisoned they pose no threat. After punishment they can be prevented from returning to the practice of psychotherapy for at least the length of their criminal justice sentence by making that prohibition a condition of their probation or parole.

Crime Victims' Assistance

As a result of passage of a criminal statute, many abused patients become eligible for money dedicated to the assistance of crime victims.

Although these funds vary in their availability and are essentially non-existent in some states, where available they can be used to finance needed treatment programs for victims. In addition, as Minnesota has done, moneys from federal criminal justice programs can be used to support educational and outreach programs designed to prevent sexual exploitation from occurring (Sanderson 1989).

Effect on Licensure

A criminal conviction would be a way to force a slow-moving medical licensure board to act, as convictions for criminal offenses such as sexual misconduct provide grounds in and of themselves for license revocation.

Arguments Against Criminalization

Remedies Already Exist

Although the present system could clearly be improved, as discussed below, functional remedies are currently in place. First, states already have laws that prohibit sexual abuse of patients, such as rape, statutory rape, indecent assault, and fraud to obtain consent to sex. These laws cover the more blatant and egregious cases, such as use of medication or electroconvulsive therapy to reduce resistance to sexual advances (see Jorgenson et al. 1991, pp. 665–666). Some states also forbid taking sexual advantage of the mentally disabled. Second, the threat of a civil lawsuit with its attendant publicity, legal costs, and potential award of monetary damages, is not inconsequential. The defense of these lawsuits is being made increasingly difficult by laws that make sex with patients negligence per se, and insurers are excluding coverage for damage awards. Third, the effect of informal peer disapproval should not be underestimated. Negative publicity and the loss of reputation, hospital privileges, referral sources, and access to academic settings of power and prestige are powerful disincentives. Current remedies appear to be having some effect. Although the results are not conclusive, a trend toward a declining rate of sexual involvement with patients has been noted (Pope et al. 1993, p. 284).

Obscuring the Issue

Sexual abuse of patients is underreported now, and criminalization may further decrease the reporting rate. Although psychiatrists have an ethical duty to report unprofessional behavior, and many states have enacted mandatory reporting statutes (Strasburger et al. 1990), psychiatrists who discover a patient has been exploited may be unwilling to report a colleague if an ethics or licensing board complaint would lead to criminal prosecution. Many patients, as part of their trauma, are still trying to protect an abusive therapist. Trapped by their ambivalence, they are often reluctant to subject their therapist to the jeopardy of a criminal conviction.

Malpractice Coverage

When a therapist's sexual misconduct results in a criminal conviction, the victim may be deprived of damages awarded in a subsequent civil lawsuit. Most malpractice insurance policies cover only negligent acts, not intentional or criminal acts, and the personal assets of the therapist may be inadequate to pay the damage award. After a criminal prosecution a victim may win a civil suit only to have the therapist's insurer assert that it is not liable to pay the damages awarded by the jury. This issue has not been widely contested because of the limited number of criminal convictions to date. There is some precedent that insurers may be required to pay civil damages, even in states where the misconduct has been criminalized (*Vigilant Insurance Co. v. Kambly*).

Admission of Guilt

The risk of criminal prosecution will substantially reduce the likelihood that an offending psychiatrist will admit misbehavior. Offenders will invoke fifth-amendment rights against self-incrimination, which will impede the process of discovery and lessen the likelihood of settlement in civil cases until the criminal trial is completed. "Taking the fifth" may also hinder the procedures of ethics committees and licensure boards. Psychiatrists who might wish to apologize and make amends will be much less likely to do so. This is unfortunate, as a simple apology often does much to help a victim heal, yet an apology is much less likely to be forthcoming if it would produce evidence against the psychiatrist at a criminal trial.

Victims' Loss of Control

Some victim advocates think that filing a criminal complaint helps a victim regain the sense of control that is so often lost following abuse. Whether the feeling of being in control of life is greater following a criminal complaint than after filing a civil lawsuit or a complaint to a licensing board has not been demonstrated. Victims, moreover, do not control the process of a criminal trial; a victim can halt the process by deciding not to testify, but otherwise control is in the hands of the prosecutor, whose decisions determine how the case is pursued.

Deterrence Unproved

Common sense and anecdotal information suggest that criminalization will deter the sexual exploitation of patients, but the hypothesis has yet to be confirmed empirically. Although it may be that as a growing number of states choose to pass criminal statutes, and more criminal convictions are publicized, it will be possible to demonstrate a connection with a reduced prevalence of abuse. To date, however, even though criminalization laws have been enacted, too few criminal charges have actually been filed to analyze a trend.

Lack of Rehabilitation

None of the criminalization statutes passed so far contain any provision for rehabilitation of offenders. Although this is a pathway that licensure boards can follow in dealing with impaired physicians, conviction of a felony in most states will simply lead to loss of medical license. Some offenders may be nontreatable individuals, but others may be depressed or have a disorder that, if treated, would restore them to social usefulness. Society, as well as the individual, has an investment in a medical education. A social policy treating these people as hopelessly unredeemable criminals may not be the best way to deal with this asset.

Consent and Sexism

Most criminalization statutes specifically exclude the defense of consent by the patient. The exclusion creates a strict liability for the therapist similar to that of statutory rape. If the behavior has been enacted, then the crime has been committed. Some critics believe that these statutes stigmatize female patients as "presumptive sillies" (Leff 1967) who are incompetent to give consent. Eliminating the defense of consent appears to imply that women are always incapable of dealing equally with men in a professional-client relationship.

In answering this criticism, it must be remembered that there is a power imbalance that is essential to sexual exploitation, and it flows from the therapist's professional status. Therapists have particular knowledge, training, and experience upon which even a sophisticated patient, male or female, must rely. Like rape, sexual exploitation is an abuse of power, and it is not limited to a match of male therapist and female patient. The public often overlooks the fact that male patients are also harmed by sexual exploitation, suffering similar symptoms to those experienced by women.

Consent becomes irrelevant and the issue of sexism disappears when the psychiatrist-patient relationship is considered as a fiduciary relationship. As fiduciary, the doctor is party to a relationship of special trust, like that of a trustee. A fiduciary must perform his or her role with an especially high standard of behavior, "a duty to act primarily for another's benefit," maintaining "scrupulous good faith and candor" (Black 1968, p. 753). A patient can have confidence that the doctor will stay in his or her professional role because of this special relationship. The vulnerability of patients seeking treatment is protected by the doctor's duty to maintain role boundaries, to attend only to patient needs, and to do no harm. Since the sole responsibility of maintaining these role boundaries of the treatment rests with the doctor, not with the patient, attention should focus entirely on the therapist's behavior, not on that of the patient.

Professional Unfairness

Many believe that criminalization places an undue burden on the already overregulated profession of psychiatry and stigmatizes psychiatrists unfairly. Some feel that it is simply unfair to invoke criminal penalties for one kind of professional relationship while not penalizing sexual behavior in other forms of fiduciary relationship, such as teacher-student, attorney-client, guardian-ward, and trustee-beneficiary. Sexual contact within the medical doctor–medical patient relationship has been criminalized only to the extent that it falls within the ambit of statutes covering rape or fraud. The legal profession, however, is beginning to focus on the issue of sexual exploitation of its clients, and other exploitations of special trust relationships, such as insider trading, have been prohibited by law and made subject to criminal penalties.

Model Criminal Statute

In 8 of the 14 states that have criminalized psychotherapist-patient sex, the legislation was supported by the local district branch of the American Psychiatric Association (APA). The APA itself has not taken an official position either to advocate or to disapprove of such legislation, but the APA's Council on Psychiatry and Law has prepared a resource document to assist district branches in their deliberations over the issue (Council on Psychiatry and Law 1993; Hoge et al.1993). The document recognizes "the differing perspectives and actual experiences of psychiatrists [that] may account for the diversity of views among district branches regarding the necessity of criminal sanctions." For groups that decide to support criminalization, the document offers the following model criminalization statute:

Section 1. Definitions

Mental Health Professional.   In this Act, "mental health professional" includes psychiatrists, other physicians, and other persons who render or offer to render services for the purpose of assessing, diagnosing, or treating emotional, mental, or behavioral disorders, or who offer services to alleviate problems pertaining to interpersonal relationships, work and life adjustment, and personal effectiveness which are caused by mental or emotional disorders or distress. This Act pertains to mental health professionals who are licensed and unlicensed, and to mental health professionals in training.

   Patient.   In this Act, "patient" is defined as a person who obtains a professional consultation, or who obtains an assessment, diagnostic, or therapeutic service from a mental health professional.

Sexual Penetration.   In this Act, "sexual penetration" means sexual intercourse, cunnilingus, fellatio, anal intercourse, or any intrusion, however slight, into the genital or anal openings of the patient's body of any part of the mental health professional's body or any object used by the mental health professional for this purpose. Emission of semen is not a required element of "sexual penetration."

Indecent Sexual Contact.   In this Act, "indecent sexual conduct" means intentional touching by the mental health professional, or by the patient with the cooperation or consent of the mental health profession-al, of the genitals, anus, or the immediately surrounding areas, including the groin, inner thighs and buttocks, or the breasts, or the clothing cov-ering any of these areas of the other person, other than in accordance with practices generally recognized as legitimate by the mental health profession.

Sexual Misconduct.   In this Act, "sexual misconduct" means either sexual penetration or indecent sexual contact.

Section 2. Punishment for Sexual Misconduct

(a) A mental health professional who engages in sexual misconduct with a patient during the period that a professional relationship exists between the mental health professional and the patient, or who termi-nates a professional relationship with a patient primarily for the purpose of engaging in sexual misconduct and who thereafter engages in sexual misconduct with the patient shall be convicted of a felony and shall be punished as provided in paragraph (c).

(b) The consent of the patient to sexual misconduct shall not be a de-fense in a prosecution under this section.

(c) A first offense in violation of this Section shall be punished by a term of imprisonment not exceeding xx years unless the sexual miscon-duct included one or more acts of sexual penetration, in which case the term of imprisonment may not exceed yy years. A second or subsequent offense may be punished by a term of imprisonment not exceeding zz years.

Section 3. Shielding of Records

That portion of the records of the court or any police department of the state or any of its political subdivisions, which contains the name of the patient involved in an alleged offense prohibited by this Act in any docu-ments relating to arrest, investigation, complaint or indictment for such an offense, shall be withheld from public inspection [as provided in the state's "rape shield" law].

Among the 14 states that have enacted statutes, 13 have made sexual misconduct a felony, and 1 has made it a misdemeanor. Consent is no defense in 12 of the 14. The statutes apply to all licensed mental health practitioners (psychiatrists, psychologists, social workers) as well as other individuals who purport to perform or provide psychotherapy. The maximum penalties imposed range from 1 to 18 years imprisonment and fines range from $5,000 to $15,000. (Fines under the Colorado statute range from $2,000 to $500,000.)

Reporting Statutes

To enable action by licensure boards and criminal prosecutors, a number of states have enacted mandatory reporting statutes. These statutes create a duty for a subsequently treating psychotherapist who learns of sexual exploitation of a patient by a mental health professional to report that abuse (Strasburger et al. 1990). These requirements seek both to identify sanction offenders who have exploited patients and to decrease the potential for abusing other patients in the future.

Reporting statutes must be carefully drawn to avoid retraumatizing those who have been victimized (Gartrell et al. 1987). For a variety of reasons victims may wish not to publicly identify those who have abused them—or perhaps not at first. Forcing them to do so prematurely aggravates feelings of being helpless and out of control and retraumatizes them. Forced reporting also undermines the trust, so difficult to reestablish after victimization, that information given to a subsequently treating therapist will be kept confidential. Because treatment may be threatened by reporting against the will of the patient, reporting should be mandatory for the therapist only when the patient gives permission.

Sex With Former Patients

Although the American Psychiatric Association has now declared that sex with former patients is unethical, 12 of the 14 existing criminal statutes cover at most the 2 years after the termination of psychother-apy. (Iowa and Minnesota forbid sex with former patients forever if the patient remains emotionally dependent on the therapist.) Some feel that criminalization of romantic relationships long after the profes-sional relationship has ended represents an inappropriate, invasive en-croachment on personal freedom and decision making, especially if the professional contact was circumscribed and brief, and also belittles for-mer patients. It is uncertain whether criminalization of sexual contact long after treatment will pass constitutional muster; privacy rights and freedom of association may prevail in this area. Although it is argued that transference is enduring and therefore so is its potential for abuse ("once a patient, always a patient"), at some point the potential for harm seems likely to become remote, or at least as unlikely as the harm inherent in most "ordinary" sexual relationships (Appelbaum and Jorgenson 1991).

Discussion

Does criminalization go too far? Is a psychiatrist-patient sexual rela-tionship sufficiently harmful to justify imposing criminal as opposed to lesser "professional" penalties? For example, abandonment, which may cause harm and lead to penalties through a civil lawsuit, does not give rise to criminal prosecution. Even negligence that is found to lead di-rectly to suicide is not punished by criminal penalties.

Where current disciplinary procedures are ineffective, there is reason to remedy the defects in the current system of sanctions and deterrents rather than create new crimes. In the furor over psychotherapist-patient sex, a misperception that there are no current remedies has led to overlooking the potential of strengthening the remedies that already exist. Statutes creating civil causes of action that establish, as a matter of law, that sexual misconduct is negligence per se will facilitate the prosecution of civil lawsuits. In these suits the negligence per se creates an irrebuttable presumption about the therapist's duty of care (Jorgenson et al. 1991, p. 702). Likewise, lengthening the statute of limitations, or tolling the statute until the discovery of harm, would re-move an obstacle to civil suits (Jorgenson and Appelbaum 1991).

The problem of unlicensed therapists may be dealt with through licensure to practice psychotherapy, registration laws, and laws permitting injunctive relief. Licensure laws require the fulfillment of standards in order to practice psychotherapy. Revocation of license or registration can halt the practice of offending therapists. At present only Florida requires a license to practice psychotherapy, and registration is required only by Colorado and Minnesota. In states where unlicensed, unregistered psychotherapists are permitted to practice, injunctive relief can bar therapists who have abused patients (Colorado 1988). The statute can specify that if a mental health professional has lost his or her license to practice (or never had one), on application by a district attorney, a licensing board, or the patient/victim, a court may issue an order enjoining the continuation of practice. Failure to observe the injunction would result in prosecution for contempt of court.

Statutes that establish employer liability for sexually exploitative psychotherapists encourage both screening and monitoring of mental health employees and thereby increase the public's protection. Outlawing silence agreements for offenders who have settled civil lawsuits enables both public and professional scrutiny of their practices. The recently enacted National Data Bank legislation strikes at these silence agreements.

Education of both patients and psychotherapists can be expected to raise consciousness about this issue and effectively reduce the frequency of future abuses. The publicity attendant on high-profile cases of abuse has been salutary in increasing both public and professional awareness (Noel and Watterson 1992). In California, the reporting statute requires psychotherapists to provide information to exploited patients as to the criminal, civil, ethical, and regulatory options open to them, and how to proceed to initiate the process of complaint (California 1990). Unfortunately, this intervention reaches only patients who go on to treatment with a subsequent psychotherapist; many who have been harmed are unable to form another trusting therapeutic relationship. Education of trainees and practitioners about the issue has received increased professional attention (American Psychiatric Association 1986, 1990; Edelwich and Brodsky 1991; Pope et al. 1993; Strasburger et al. 1992). The APA has undertaken the development of special programs to teach residents and practitioners about sexual misconduct and has sponsored workshops and symposia at annual and district branch meetings. These efforts to inform both professionals and the public must be continued.

Criminalization continues to be a complex and controversial matter. A crime is an offense against the state, and labeling psychotherapist sexual misconduct a crime indicates a sense that the effects of the behavior extend beyond individuals to the collective public. Patient harm and professional standards are certainly central to the debate, but the strength of these legitimate concerns has been amplified by media hyperbole—sex is always a sexy issue. Sexual politics further pressure our public wisdom. We are moved too quickly by the cry, "There oughta be a law." Declaring social problems to be criminal does not necessarily eliminate them.

A pause before rushing to enact new laws is justified by more than professional defensiveness. As society's last line of defense, criminalization should not be undertaken lightly. Careful consideration must be given to the decision to initiate penalties that are society's strongest way to formally condemn human behavior (Barker 1990, p. 1280). Clinical, ethical, and legal issues deserve thoughtful consideration when deciding whether criminalization is an appropriate social policy.

References

Arizona: Ariz Rev Stat Ann (1996)

American Psychiatric Association: Ethical Concerns About Sexual Involvement Between Psychiatrists and Patients (videotape). Washington, DC, American Psychiatric Press, 1986

American Psychiatric Association: Reporting Ethical Concerns About Sexual Involvement Between Psychiatrists and Patients (videotape). Washington, DC, American Psychiatric Press, 1990

Appelbaum P, Jorgenson L: Psychotherapist-patient sexual contact after termination of treatment: an analysis and a proposal. Am J Psychiatry 148:1466–1473, 1991

Barker JA: Professional-client sex: is criminal liability an appropriate means of enforcing professional responsibility? UCLA Law Review 40:1275–1339, 1990

Bass A: Licenses revoked, therapists still practicing. Boston Globe, July 6, 1993, p 1

Black HC: Black's Law Dictionary, 4th Edition. St. Paul, MN, West Publishing, 1968

Bouhoutsos J, Holroyd J, Lerman H, et al: Sexual intimacy between psycho-
    therapists and patients. Professional Psychology, Research and Practice
    14:185, 1983
California: Cal Business and Prof Code § 337 (West 1990)
California: Cal Business and Prof Code § 729 (West 1993)
Colorado: Colo Rev Stat § 12–43–708 (Supp 1988)
Colorado: Colo Rev Stat § 18–3–405.5 (1992)
Connecticut: Substitute House Bill No. 6437 Public Act No 93340 (effective
    Oct 1, 1993)
Council on Psychiatry and Law, American Psychiatric Association: Resource
    Document: Legal Sanctions for Mental Health Professional–Patient Sex.
    Washington, DC, American Psychiatric Association, 1993
Edelwich J, Brodsky A: Sexual Dilemmas for the Helping Professional. New
    York, Brunner/Mazel, 1991
Epstein RS: Keeping Boundaries, Maintaining Safety and Integrity in the
    Psychotherapeutic Process. Washington, DC, American Psychiatric Press,
    1994, p 3
Florida: Fla Stat Ann § 491.0111–491.0112 (West 1993)
Gabbard G (ed): Sexual Exploitation in Professional Relationships. Washing-
    ton, DC, American Psychiatric Press, 1989
Gartrell N, Herman J, Olarte S, et al: Reporting practices of psychiatrists who
    knew of sexual misconduct by colleagues. Am J Orthopsychiatry 57:289–
    293, 1987
Georgia: Ga Code Ann § 16–6–5.1 (1992)
Hoge SK, Jorgenson L, Goldstein N, et al: Mental health professional–patient
    sexual misconduct: legal sanctions. A resource document of the American
    Psychiatric Association. Approved May 1993. Bulletin of the American
    Academy of Psychiatry and the Law, 1993
Iowa: Iowa Code Ann § 709.15 (West 1992)
Jorgenson L, Appelbaum P: For whom the statute tolls: extending the time
    during which patients can sue. Hospital and Community Psychiatry 42:
    683–684, 1991
Jorgenson L, Randles R, Strasburger L: The furor over psychotherapist-
    patient sexual contact: new solutions to an old problem. William and
    Mary Law Review 32:645–732, 1991
Leff AA: Unconscionability and the code—the emperor's new clause. Univer-
    sity of Pennsylvania Law Review 115:485–559, 1967
Maine: ME Rev Stat Ann tit 17-A, § 253 (2) (I) (1992)
Masters WH, Johnson VA: Principles of the new sex therapy. Am J Psychiatry
    133:548, 1976

Minnesota: Minn Stat Ann § 609.341 et seq (West 1993)

New Hampshire: NH Rev Stat Ann 623-A:1 et seq (1992)

New Mexico: NM Stat Ann § 30–9–10 through 30–9–16 (effective 1993)

Noel B, Watterson K: You Must Be Dreaming. New York: Poseidon, 1992

North Dakota: ND Cent Code § 12.1–20–06.1 (1991)

Pope KS: Therapist-patient sex syndrome: a guide for attorneys and subsequent therapists to assessing damage, in Sexual Exploitation in Professional Relationships. Edited by Gabbard G. Washington, DC, American Psychiatric Press, 1989, pp 40–45

Pope KS: Sexual Involvement with Therapists: Patient Assessment, Subsequent Therapy, Forensics. Washington, DC, American Psychological Association, 1994, pp 6–7

Pope KS, Bouhoutsos JC: Sexual Intimacy Between Therapists and Patients. New York, Praeger, 1986

Pope KS, Levenson H, Schover L: Sexual intimacy in psychology training: results and implications of a national survey. Am Psychol 34:682–689, 1979

Pope KS, Sonne JL, Holroyd J: Sexual Feelings in Psychotherapy. Washington, DC, American Psychological Association, 1993

Riley v Presnell 565 NE2d 780 (Mass 1991)

Roy v Hartogs, 366 NYS2d 297 (1975)

Sanderson B (ed): It's Never OK: A Handbook for Professionals on Sexual Exploitation by Counselors and Therapists. St. Paul, MN, Minnesota Department of Corrections, 1989

South Dakota: Senate Bill 236 (Enacted 1993)

Storring V, Zaritsky J (producers): Frontline: My Doctor, My Lover. Washington, DC, Public Broadcasting System, 1991

Strasburger LH, Jorgenson L, Randles R: Mandatory reporting of sexually exploitative psychotherapists. Bulletin of the American Academy of Psychiatry and the Law 18:379–384, 1990

Strasburger LH, Jorgenson L, Randles R: Criminalization of psychotherapist-patient sex. Am J Psychiatry 148:859–863, 1991

Strasburger LH, Jorgenson L, Sutherland P: The prevention of psychotherapist sexual misconduct: avoiding the slippery slope. Am J Psychother 46:544–555, 1992

Texas: Senate Bill 210 (enacted May 22, 1993)

Utah: Utah Code Ann § 76–5–406 (12) (1998)

Vigilant Insurance Co. v Kambly, 114 Mich App 683, 319 NW2d 382 (1992)

Wisconsin: Wis Stat Ann § 940.22 (2) (West 1992)

3

INSURANCE COVERAGE FOR UNDUE FAMILIARITY
Law, Policy, and Economic Reality

Alan A. Stone, M.D., and
Duncan C. MacCourt, J.D.

O ver the past 30 years, state and federal courts have struggled with the question of whether malpractice insurance does or should cover sexual contact between mental health practitioners and their patients. These troubling and sometimes sordid narratives of sexual exploitation, along with the legal questions they raise, merit scrutiny, but by no means do they reveal the whole complicated insurance story. The relevant cases are generally the product of lawsuits that arose when insurance companies raised technical legal objections to providing coverage to mental health practitioners who were sued for sexual misconduct —or, as it is often called in insurance policies, "undue familiarity." The judges were called on to decide the scope of coverage by interpreting the contractual language in the malpractice policies. When the insurance companies began to lose these cases, they adopted a variety of

37

strategies to rewrite insurance policies, to include caps and exclusions on undue familiarity, and to change their business practices. In this chapter we therefore describe some of the equally important transactions and dealings taking place outside the reported cases in the hope of conveying a more comprehensive account of this complex and interesting intersection of law, morality, and malpractice insurance. Appendix 3–1 contains citations to and summaries of many of the reported cases regarding insurability of sexual misconduct by both therapists and nontherapists. It provides a useful, chronological overview of this expanding area of the law of vital concern to medical professionals.

Malpractice insurance coverage is of course critical to medical professionals who might otherwise be financially ruined by a major lawsuit. But coverage is also essential to the victims of sexual exploitation if they are to be able to seek vindication and compensation in a civil action. The professional's malpractice insurer provides the funds—often called the "deep pocket"—out of which come the monetary compensation for the victim and the money to pay her contingency-fee lawyer, her expert witnesses, and her other legal expenses.[1] In addition, many malpractice plaintiffs seek some form of punitive damages, which the court may impose on the malfeasor to punish him and which are assessed over and above compensatory damages.[2] These awards can be very large, amounting to hundreds of thousands of dollars.[3] Although a small number of offending psychotherapists have enough personal wealth to constitute a deep pocket of their own even without liability insurance, most certainly do not. Plaintiffs' contingency-fee lawyers describe such uninsured defendants as being virtually judgment proof, for even in an "open-and-shut" case there would be no remuneration for the lawyers who represent the victim in a lawsuit. The existence of medical malpractice insurance provides the monetary incentive for the victim's case to be heard in a court of law: it provides, in a very practical sense, the means by which the patient obtains an advocate through which she can tell her story.[4]

The recent decisions of liability insurance providers to close the deep pocket by excluding or capping coverage for undue familiarity must surely have had a significant impact on victim litigation and compensation. Such limits on the amount that can be recovered in a malpractice suit operate to dissuade attorneys from taking cases and plaintiffs from filing suit. At the same time, however, victims now seem more determined to press their claims, and plaintiffs' lawyers have become increasingly hungry for clients as the oversupply of lawyers seems at last to have had an impact on the demand for their services. And even in the face of such explicit insurance caps and exclusions of coverage for undue familiarity, there has emerged a small group of plaintiffs' lawyers interested in this very narrow and specialized area. They seem as confident that they can get around the insurance barriers that have been erected as the insurers are that they cannot. As this chapter was being prepared, both sides were still claiming victory. It is their battles that produced the legal opinions that form the substance of this chapter.

Background to the Controversy

During the 1970s it seemed that insuring mental health professionals for malpractice liability might be a profitable enterprise. Psychiatry, for example, was a low-risk profession compared to almost every other medical specialty. Rates for the American Psychiatric Association (APA)–sponsored malpractice insurance were set at three-quarters of the prevailing rate for the lowest-risk general practitioners. Even at that low premium rate, however, the cash reserves held by the insurance companies began to accumulate because malpractice claims against psychiatrists were so infrequent. The APA's for-profit insurer, Chubb Associates, seemed to be sitting on a gold mine, for such reserves can earn substantial amounts of money for the insurance company. The APA therefore decided in the early 1980s to form its own nonprofit liability insurance company—what is informally called a "bedpan" insurer[5]—in the expectation of recouping some of this windfall profit and reducing its members' premiums. Based on its favorable actuarial experience over several decades, the APA introduced with great fanfare low-premium malpractice policies for psychiatrists. Unfortunately, the timing could not have been much worse: malpractice claims, lawsuits, and damage awards began to escalate dramatically in the 1980s, and the suits with the most significant damage awards were suits for undue familiarity. Faced with these escalating awards, the APA's newly formed bedpan insurer barely staved off bankruptcy and was forced to raise its premiums, much to the dismay of its membership. Despite some opposition from members who were concerned about the consequences for

abused patients, the APA eventually resolved to exclude claims of undue familiarity by rewriting the contractual terms of its insurance
policy.

Other mental health professionals (e.g., psychoanalysts, psychologists, social workers, and lower-echelon practitioners) had been insured for even lower premiums. They experienced the same pattern of
rapidly increasing claims of undue familiarity. A similar pattern was
seen in the clergy and other helping professions. Undue familiarity rapidly became the most important cause of successful malpractice cases
against psychologists covered by the APA-sponsored plan. And damage
awards were high: a single case against a psychologist reportedly paid
$2.3 million.[6] As a result of such high awards, some insurers discontin-
ued their malpractice policies. According to one disgruntled psychologist, "We are the only profession dropped by our insurance carrier
because of the frequency of malpractice suits involving sexual impro-
prieties."[7] The crisis of public confidence that confronted these professional organizations and the solvency crisis that confronted the APA's
strapped liability insurers now set off a debate: Should undue familiarity be covered by association-sponsored insurance plans? The arguments reprised a long-standing controversy in tort law, of which
professional malpractice is a component. The controversy has two dimensions, one definitional and the other ethical and moral.

Legal Definitions of Malpractice

The particular language of the liability insurance contract will determine the outcome of a dispute about the insurability of sexual misconduct, because that is the text the court will be called on to interpret.
Here we consider the standard or generic policy contract initially issued
to mental health professionals at a time when the insurance companies
had not yet focused on the necessity of capping or excluding claims
based on undue familiarity. These generic policies often contained language such as the following:

> The insurer will pay all sums which the insured shall become legally ob-
> ligated to pay as damages arising out of the performance of professional
> services rendered or which should have been rendered during the policy
> period of the insured . . . and the company shall have the right and duty

to defend him in his name and on his behalf any suit against the insured alleging damages, even if such suit is groundless, false, or fraudulent.[8]

As an initial matter, one might argue that undue familiarity between a physician and his or her patient is an activity completely outside the realm of providing professional services as contemplated in these generic malpractice policies. Such definitional arguments have successfully been made by insurers in the case of dentists who have sexually molested their patients; although the dentist may be personally responsible for harming his patient and liable for any damages he causes, his sexual abuse of a patient is quite outside the realm of practicing dentistry or providing dental services.[9] (Note that insurance contracts and cases use the words *providing, rendering,* and *furnishing* interchangeably.) Therefore, by definition such behavior would not be dental malpractice and would not be covered by a generic professional malpractice policy. However, even this apparently straightforward distinction is difficult to maintain when one considers the circumstances and nature of much sexual abuse.

Consider, for example, the dentist who tells his patient that nitrous oxide anesthesia is required to care for her teeth and then, having rendered her stuporous, sexually molests her. Or the family doctor who, having anesthetized a young male patient for a minor procedure, then sexually abuses him. Certainly both the dentist and the family doctor are grossly unethical and guilty of a criminal offense, but since the misconduct occurred during the provision of anesthesia, it might also be considered professional malpractice. The claim of malpractice is even more compelling if the anesthesia itself caused some harmful effect to the patient such as brain damage. Unfortunately, these awful examples are taken from actual cases as judges struggled to draw lines between what was and was not the provision of services and therefore within the realm of professional malpractice.[10]

This definitional line drawing has been much less difficult in mental health cases. Despite the insurers' arguments that undue familiarity is not a professional service covered by the generic policy language, many courts have held that sexual contact with a patient constitutes negligent delivery of professional services. Beginning with the landmark case of *Zipkin v. Freeman,*[11] the courts have developed a coherent rationale for finding negligence, basing their decisions on the recognized presence during psychotherapy of the transference-countertransference phenomenon. In such cases, courts have determined that a central feature of providing psychotherapy is the management of the transference-countertransference; therefore, the occurrence of any undue familiarity is construed as professional malpractice since it derives from the therapist's mismanagement of the phenomenon.[12]

The same sexual misconduct by a general practitioner or a surgeon would not be so considered, however. For example, courts are unlikely to determine that the surgeon who arranges to meet a patient in a hotel room to have sex is engaged in behavior covered by his malpractice policy, because there exists no recognized transference-countertransference phenomenon that is the surgeon's professional responsibility to manage. Similarly, the general practitioner who engages in sexual conduct in his office is unlikely to be covered, regardless of whether or not the patient consents.[13] Although the physicians' behavior in these circumstances may be deemed unethical and reprehensible—as is the mental health professional's—only the latter's behavior counts under the definition of providing professional services.

Typical of such decisions is *Vigilant Insurance Co. v. Employers Insurance of Wausau,* in which a psychiatrist's insurer brought an action seeking a contribution for a malpractice settlement from the psychiatrist's other insurer.[14] The psychiatrist had engaged in nude "primal therapy" sessions with one patient and had engaged in sexual intercourse during one of these sessions.[15] The psychiatrist had also ordered another patient, "as her physician," to disrobe and remain at his apartment.[16] The psychiatrist had been issued a standard malpractice policy that covered "injury or death resulting from rendering or failing to render . . . professional services by the insured . . . performed in the practice of the insured's profession."[17] In holding that the nonsettling insurer was required to contribute to the settlement, a federal district court determined that, "in light of the transference phenomenon . . . the acts of which [the former patients] complained were sufficiently related to therapy to fall within the coverage of the insurance policies."[18] Similarly, in *St. Paul Fire and Marine Insurance Company v. Love,* the Minnesota Supreme Court stated that "where the transference phenomenon pervades the therapeutic alliance . . . the patient's claim results from the providing of improper professional services or the withholding of proper services."[19]

In this line of cases, therefore, the presence of the transference phenomenon in the psychotherapist-patient relationship makes all the difference between an insurer's liability and the insured practitioner being forced to cover a judgment or settlement himself. Although the language of the different cases varies and suggests that coverage is not universally applicable to mental health professionals in all circumstances, an analysis of reported decisions reveals that professional services covered by generic policies invariably include sexual misconduct if the practitioner is providing any form of psychotherapy.[20, 21] As one court stated,

> a sexual relationship between the therapist and patient cannot be viewed separately from the therapeutic relationship that has developed between them. The transference phenomenon makes it impossible that the patient will have the same emotional response to sexual contact with the therapist that he or she would have to sexual contact with other persons.[22]

The same logic applies to all mental health professionals. Crucial to these decisions is the idea that, because the transference phenomenon is an accepted part of treatment, the mishandling of transference by a therapist is no different from the mishandling of a surgical technique or a misprescription of drugs.[23] Basically, the psychiatrist, psychologist, and social worker are seen to wield the transference phenomenon as a part of their therapeutic armamentarium in the same way that the family doctor wields penicillin for the treatment of streptococcus and the general surgeon wields the scalpel. The mishandling of the transference therefore becomes, as the *Love* court has stated, an "occupational risk" that is covered by the standard language "professional services rendered or which should have been rendered."[24] (The Minnesota Supreme Court later appeared to limit this approach, stating that the existence of the transference and its mishandling will not be presumed just because a psychotherapist is involved; rather, the determination must be developed by expert testimony.[25])

Critics of this legal line drawing have noted that the transference phenomenon can be present in many other doctor-patient relationships, not just that of the psychiatrist and patient. Minnesota Supreme Court Justice Coyne's dissent in *St. Paul Fire and Marine Insurance Company v. Love*, for example, illustrates the feeling that insurers for mental health professionals are being made to bear a special burden because psychotherapists are being mistakenly viewed as existing apart from other medical specialties:

> [I]t is certainly not unheard of for a patient to fall in love with a surgeon who has relieved a physical problem or a family doctor or gynecologist or lawyer consulted in regard to marital problems. Neither is it unheard of for the physician or the lawyer to fall in love with the patient. I am un-aware of the conduct of any of those professionals having been charac-terized as "the mishandling of the transference phenomenon" or succumbing to an occupational hazard. Until now, such circumstances have always been recognized for what they are—conduct removed from the professional relationship.[26]

In interpreting standard policies covering professional services, however, courts have generally rejected this argument by focusing on the unique nature of the psychotherapeutic encounter. Although trans-ference undoubtedly does occur between professionals who do not provide mental health services and their clients, these courts employ classic psychoanalytic grounds to reason that in no other medical spe-cialty is the presence of the transference phenomenon an accepted part of the treatment that the mental health practitioner must employ if he or she is to effect a cure of the patient's psychological disorder.[27]

The courts also take an expansive view of the sexual boundary viola-tions, refusing to focus only on cases in which the sexual act occurs in the office or during a psychotherapy session. If a sexual act occurs dur-ing therapy, or outside of therapy but between a psychiatrist and his pa-tient, the insurer is likely to be forced to indemnify the psychiatrist. For example, one court has found coverage under a standard policy cover-ing professional services when a therapist hugged a patient during a therapy session and progressed to kissing her during their visits, but did not engage in the most damaging sexual contact until after the ter-mination of therapy.[28] In fact, the termination of therapy only to have a sexual relationship commence, develop, or continue is a fairly common scenario in these cases.[29] Although terminating therapy in these cir-cumstances was at one time considered ethical, it will no longer be deemed to end the doctor-patient relationship and will not preclude liability for undue familiarity. In fact, it may lead to additional types of negligence claims such as failure to refer, failure to consult, and abandonment.

This transference-oriented definition of rendering, providing, or furnishing professional services can encompass a wide variety of boundary violations not confined to sexual activity with the patient. In one sordid North Carolina case, for example, a patient found his psychiatrist in bed with his wife.[30] Expert testimony established that the psychiatrist had violated his ethical and professional duties to his patient.[31] A substantial jury award with punitive damages was given at trial.[32] On appeal, the psychiatrist's lawyers tried to argue that this unethical and unprofessional behavior did not occur during the furnishing of professional services. The court swept aside the definitional argument, stating, "Special duties exist in the practice of medicine not to ruin a doctor and patient relationship, and those duties are *more critical in psychiatry* than in other areas of medicine."[33]

Ethical and Moral Dimensions: Intentional Acts and Public Policy

Although the courts have concluded that such sexual misconduct as previously described is malpractice, at least under their interpretation of the generic policy language, one can understand that an insurance company might want to argue that they are nonetheless not required to indemnify such "intentional," "willful," "wanton," and even criminal behavior. In fact, many medical malpractice policies contain exclusions for intentional and/or criminal acts; however, in cases involving psychotherapists the courts have often found that the sexual misconduct is still not excluded.[34]

Insurers often argue that undue familiarity may fall within the legal interpretation of the language of an insurance contract, but as a matter of *public policy* malpractice insurance should not cover the sexual exploitation of emotionally vulnerable patients. This argument views professional insurance as protecting and indemnifying the practitioner from his negligence, understood as unintentional acts or omissions, and not from *intentional* acts amounting to malfeasance such as sexual misconduct.

The concept of intentionality is of central importance in law, and various meanings have been given to it. At some basic level, all of us distinguish between intentional and unintentional acts: Oliver Wendell Holmes opined that even a dog can tell the difference between being kicked and being tripped over.[35] This moral intuition leads to a legal distinction between what the law calls intentional torts (e.g., punching someone in the nose or sexual exploitation) and unintentional torts (e.g., prescribing the wrong medication or negligence). Behind the distinction lies the idea that insurance should cover unintentional but not intentional torts; this distinction—recognized in some jurisdictions by statute, by insurance regulation, or by judicial decision—has been seized upon by insurance companies to argue against indemnification of undue familiarity.[36] But courts in some cases have been loath to accept the distinction. A New York court in 1986 concluded that a psychiatrist's insurance policy provided coverage because the psychiatrist "did not intend to injure his patients," although he intended to have sex with them.[37]

Another related public policy argument is that allowing insurance coverage would give the mental health practitioner a "license" to exploit his patients. So reasoning, Vigilant, the insurer of a psychiatrist who had sexually molested one of his patients, refused to compensate the victim under a malpractice policy that did not specifically exclude undue familiarity.[38] The company argued that it would be contrary to public policy to allow an insured who had sexually exploited his patient to "profit from his own wrong doing" or "encourage the commission of wrongful acts by relieving the wrongdoer of financial responsibility therefore."[39]

The court had no trouble rejecting the apparent logic of Vigilant's argument, for it doubted that the offending psychiatrist was "induced to engage in this conduct" or that other psychiatrists "in the future would be induced to similar misconduct" by allowing insurance coverage.[40] Nor, as the court reasoned, is it the therapist who benefits from insurance coverage but rather his "innocent victim."[41] And it is this innocent victim who has been left out of the sometimes self-righteous public policy pronouncements of the malpractice insurers. (The idea that the victim is somehow not entirely innocent because she consented or even took the initiative seems to have occurred to a few judges in the past.[42] However, in recent cases the courts generally seem even more critical of psychotherapists who become involved with sexually aggressive or seductive patients.[43])

The court in the *Vigilant* case was dealing with a generic policy that neither capped nor excluded undue familiarity.[44] It decided that, in the absence of a specific exclusion, the public policy concern about rewarding a malfeasor for his actions did not contravene the coverage of this category of negligent malpractice.[45] Subsequent to such decisions, the insurers rewrote their malpractice policies to avoid any ambiguity and to develop ironclad contractual language that would preclude all such legal questions. Some policies now contained caps on the amount of coverage available for undue familiarity, such as the policy issued to psychiatrists and neurologists by the American Home Assurance Company:

> The total limit of the Company's liability hereunder shall not exceed $25,000.00 in the aggregate for all damages with respect to the total of all claims against any insured(s) involving any actual or alleged erotic physical contact, or attempt thereat, or proposal thereof . . . .
>
> The Company shall not be obligated to undertake or continue to defend any suit or proceedings subject to the aforesaid $25,000.00 aggregate limit of liability after said $25,000.00 aggregate limit of liability has been exhausted by payment of judgments and/or settlements and/or other items included within the limits of liability.[46]

Later malpractice policies contained specific exclusions on the insurer's responsibility to indemnify a therapist for any damages arising out of undue familiarity. In the policy issued by the APA, for example, the following claims are excluded:

> . . . Any claim, damages or cause of action based in whole or in part on, or involving a claim of undue familiarity . . .
>
> . . . Any claim, damages or cause of action based in whole or in part on actual or alleged mishandling of the transference or countertransference phenomena, harassment, or abandonment, where the Participating member is alleged to have engaged in, or has engaged in, undue familiarity with the claimant. . . .[47]

Unlike capped policies, which have contained ambiguous, conflicting provisions simultaneously capping sexual misconduct and excluding all wrongful acts, these exclusionary policies exhibit no such ambiguity.

At least in theory, however, a court could overturn the most ironclad contract on public policy grounds. As a Washington state court noted, "The term 'public policy' . . . embraces all acts or contracts which tend clearly to injure the public health, the public morals, the public confidence in the purity of the administration of the law, or to undermine that sense of security for individual rights, whether of personal liberty or of private property, which any citizen ought to feel."[48] "Public policy is not static, but may change as the relevant factual situation and the thinking of the times change."[49]

In recent cases plaintiffs' lawyers have therefore been invoking "public policy" to challenge malpractice policies that attempted to cap or exclude coverage of undue familiarity. These cases and other plaintiff strategies are discussed below, but public policy is a "knife that cuts two ways" and can be invoked by either side of a contractual dispute. It is therefore of interest to consider further the ethical and moral—that is, the public policy—arguments against the exclusion of undue familiarity.

The premiums collected by professional liability insurance can be conceptualized not only as a fund to protect a psychotherapist, but as a victim compensation fund available for all of the patients harmed by mental health professionals. Instead of focusing on the nature of the doctor's behavior, that conception directs our attention to a different kind of question: who among those harmed by mental health professionals is more or less deserving of compensation? To exclude the group of patients, most of them women, who have been victims of sexual exploitation seems morally obtuse, particularly when one recognizes that such patients were dismissed as psychotic or silenced by convention for most of this century.[50] Indeed, one might be justly concerned that the exclusion of sexually exploited women from the victim compensation fund demonstrates that sexism and victimization of the victim continue to plague institutional policy.

There are well-crafted legal arguments that make exclusions and caps seem contrary to changing conceptions of public policy. For example, some plaintiffs' attorneys have argued that limitations on damages in cases of undue familiarity unfairly discriminate against women. Since more women than men are victims of undue familiarity,[51] the argument goes, the limitation on or exclusion of undue familiarity damages affects more women than men and therefore has what the law calls a "disparate impact" on women.[52] However, in *American Home Assur-*

ance Company v. Cohen, the Washington Supreme Court recently rejected such an argument.[53] *Cohen* involved a psychologist sued by a female patient for nine claims of malpractice, including abandonment, failure to treat competently, and mishandling of the transference.[54] The psychologist was insured by a policy that limited damages in cases of sexual misconduct to $25,000 and that capped *all* damages at that amount, whether stemming from sexual or nonsexual misconduct, if allegations of undue familiarity were raised.[55] Examining Washington state statutes, the *Cohen* court first determined that, although state law showed concern for the victims of sexual misconduct, there was no law that required compensation for victims of sexual misconduct, nor was there a statute requiring a psychologist to carry malpractice insurance.[56, 57] The court therefore determined that Washington had no public policy of compensating victims of undue familiarity through insurance coverage.[58] Furthermore, the cap did not violate a state public policy prohibiting sex discrimination because it was devised to limit the insurer's exposure to an identifiable financial risk—that is, that "a significant percentage of claims against psychologists are based on sexual misconduct."[59] (In the same case in a federal district court, American Home cited statistics that "sexual misconduct claims were the single highest category of claims filed, 20%, and resulted in 56% of proceeds paid on all claims."[60] Like the Washington Supreme Court, the federal court upheld the $25,000 cap because of "the increased risk to insurers of sexual misconduct claims."[61])

While generally upholding caps on sexual misconduct claims against both psychotherapists and other health care providers, the courts differ when evaluating the extension of the cap to all claims or causes of action. Although the *Cohen* court upheld a $25,000 cap on undue familiarity claims, it also disallowed the provision attaching this cap to all related claims.[62] The policy at question limited the entire recovery, both of sexual misconduct claims and nonsexual claims, to $25,000 if the sexual misconduct were also alleged as occurring in the "same or related course of professional treatment" as the nonsexual misconduct.[63] Furthermore, the misconduct could be alleged "at any time, either in the complaint, during discovery, at trial or otherwise."[64] The court reasoned that anyone could allege the sexual misconduct, not just the plaintiff, and therefore limit the plaintiff's recovery.[65] Such a provision provided, said the court, a clear disincentive for reporting the unethical and harmful conduct of an insured psychologist, even though such reporting would benefit the public by helping to prevent future acts of sexual misconduct in other therapeutic relationships.[66]

Examining state law, the court found a clear public policy in favor of eliminating unethical and unprofessional behavior by psychotherapists through administrative disciplinary proceedings, injunctive actions, and criminal prosecutions.[67] The court then found that the insurance provision would violate public policy by dissuading victims of sexual misconduct from "taking advantage of protective statutes aimed at stopping therapist misconduct . . . ."[68]

In contrast to *Cohen,* however, is *American Home Assurance Company v. Stone,* a federal case in which exactly the same provision was held not to violate Illinois' public policy.[69] Despite that state's "Sexual Exploitation in Therapy Act," which creates a cause of action for a patient who has been injured by a therapist's sexual misconduct,[70] the *Stone* court declined to find a public policy limiting the form or amount of coverage insurance companies can provide in cases of undue familiarity.[71]

The APA's policy contains exclusionary language indicating a similar attempt to link claims of nonsexual misconduct to undue familiarity claims. ("Any claim, damages or cause of action based in whole *or in part on, or involving* a claim of undue familiarity . . . ."[72]) Although courts have not yet considered this exclusionary language, one can expect that it will be subjected to legal challenges similar to those employed against the capped policies.

The Mechanics of Malpractice Insurance

The statistics cited above in the *Cohen* case demonstrate that, as a business matter, malpractice insurers had compelling financial reasons to limit the coverage of undue familiarity. Similarly, insurers that have contracted out of any coverage for undue familiarity claims—such as the APA's bedpan insurer—have done so out of significant financial concerns. To understand those business concerns, it is necessary to know something about the workings of liability insurance.

Professional liability insurance was traditionally provided under an "occurrence" basis. An occurrence policy for the year 1984 (a year when claims of undue familiarity escalated) would cover any malpractice liability for undue familiarity that *occurred* in that year. This means that if a therapist retired from practice at the end of 1984, he could do so with the assurance that any claims or lawsuits based on events that had *occurred* in that year would be covered by that policy. A claim of malpractice arising out of undue familiarity might be delayed several years, depending on the length of time the statute of limitations allows, and it might then take several more years for the case to be settled or go to trial for decision. However, even if the 1984 claim did not get resolved for a decade it would still be covered by the practitioner's 1984 occurrence-based policy.

This provides long-term security for the practitioner but creates what is called the "long tail" problem for the insurance company. Under an occurrence policy, the company has to maintain enough financial reserves to cover malpractice settlements and jury awards based on events that occurred as long as a decade or more before. And maintaining such reserves becomes problematic when one considers that insurers have traditionally been wary of long-term predictions of malpractice liability because new legal standards and escalating jury awards will have unexpected impact on claims resolved in future years. Actuarial estimates of the liability of mental health professionals certainly could not have anticipated a decade earlier the sudden increase that would occur in undue familiarity claims and in the large damage awards given by juries. Thus, the amount of occurrence-based premiums collected years earlier by the insurers of mental health professionals was insufficient to cover the long tail of potential damages growing out of the earlier claims.

In the 1980s this scenario threatened the financial stability of all of the companies insuring mental health professionals on an occurrence-based arrangement. As a result, these insurers found it necessary to raise their premiums, and if their policies continued to cover undue familiarity they faced the prospect of bankruptcy—a disaster for them and their members who, despite having paid their premiums, would be left with a worthless policy.

One should also recognize that bedpan insurers such as the APA's may have been unable to purchase the reinsurance they needed had they chosen to cover sexual misconduct without raising premiums astronomically. Small insurance companies protect themselves against

unexpected losses by purchasing reinsurance. In exchange for a nego-
tiated sum, the reinsurer is responsible for paying out claims if the
bedpan company exhausts all of the premiums it has collected. The reinsurer will therefore insist that the bedpan company charge an adequate premium to cover anticipated claims. But if a bedpan insurer
raises its premium by the amount necessary to cover sexual misconduct
claims, it will lose most of its members, who will look for a less expensive policy. On the other hand, the reinsurer cannot be expected to accept this kind of uncontrolled, escalating risk. From a purely business
standpoint, caps and exclusions are mechanisms to control this risk
and maintain financial stability: without them, the insurer will have a
hard time convincing a reinsurer to issue a policy.

Furthermore, bedpan insurers like the APA's have substantial obligations to the organization and its insured members. Such a company
cannot pursue business decisions that are certain to bring economic
collapse. This would have the effect of eliminating the insured member's coverage, which has been marketed as a benefit of membership in
this voluntary professional organization. The result would be to threat-
en the viability of the APA itself.

During this period, these insurance companies were also faced with
competitors who could offer mental health professionals lower-priced
malpractice premiums on a "claims-made" basis. The claims-made insurers have immediate financial advantages over the occurrence-based
companies. To illustrate, if the practitioner had purchased a less expensive claims-made policy in 1984 and no *claim* of undue familiarity was
filed in 1984, his policy for that year would have no further value, because a claims-made policy covers only claims filed *in* that year. If he
retired at the end of 1984 and the claim of undue familiarity based on
events that had occurred in 1984 was eventually filed in 1986, his 1984
claims-made policy would not indemnify him. Even in retirement he
therefore would need to keep purchasing claims-made policies each
year, or what is called a tail policy, to protect himself. This is in contrast
to an occurrence-based policy, which would cover any claim that had
occurred in 1984, regardless of when it was eventually filed. The enlightened purchaser might recognize this difference, but many will purchase the less expensive policy.

Through such claims-made policies, the insurance providers have
eliminated the long-tail problem. For business purposes, they know

much better at the end of each year where they stand because they are responsible only for claims made that year and they can calculate the likely costs to resolve them. The companies offering claims-made policies also benefit from the practitioner's prior occurrence-based policies. Thus, if the practitioner switched in 1984 from an occurrence-based to a claims-made policy, the new insurer could expect that most of the 1985 claims would be based on events that had occurred in 1984 or earlier. The occurrence-based insurer might be responsible for covering such claims, not the claims-made provider. In effect, the claims-made providers are being subsidized by the practitioner's earlier occurrence-based policies.[73] Benefiting from these financial advantages, the claims-made companies can offer substantially lower premiums. Furthermore, if they cap or exclude undue familiarity, their premiums will be even lower. Mental health practitioners, like every other consumer in the market, are susceptible to substantial price differences and can be expected to purchase policies with the lowest premiums. The vast majority will never sexually exploit a patient and need have no self-interested concern about the existence of caps and exclusions in their individual policies. Although many practitioners are concerned about victims who will go uncompensated, there is no reason to expect that these concerns will translate into a willingness to pay the much higher premiums necessary.

The problem the APA faced with its bedpan insurance company was much like the problem in ordinary health insurance wherein low-risk patients opt for lower health maintenance organization (HMO) premiums rather than remain in fee-for-service plans where they are subsidizing the sicker members of the community. The APA's bedpan insurer would have needed all of its members to agree to pay substantially higher premiums if it were to continue to cover undue familiarity. This was not about to happen. In addition, the members, despite their concerns about the victims of sexual abuse, seemed even more disturbed by the idea that insurance coverage of undue familiarity gave their unethical colleagues a license for sexual exploitation. Despite some opposition, the language of the APA's contract therefore was carefully rewritten to exclude undue familiarity and related claims. But given the economic pressures faced by insurance companies, it is remarkable that the APA's occurrence-based insurance program survived, even with this exclusion.

Indeed, the claims-made providers still market their policies with baleful warnings that practitioners who pay into occurrence-based arrangements may find that their company is bankrupt when they need the promised long-tail protection. And, as demonstrated by the *Cohen* cases, discussed above, these economic arguments are not irrelevant when a court considers invoking public policy to require an insurance company to pay claims that are excluded in the contract. If an insurance company can demonstrate, as the insurer did in *Cohen,* that limitations or exclusions are motivated by an increased risk to the company, then public policy arguments about the viability of the insurance business may prevail over concerns about disparate impact on women.

The Defendant, His Lawyer, and His Insurance Company— A Divergence of Interests

Law is like psychiatry in one important respect: problems are best understood when examined from different perspectives. It is therefore critical and useful to examine undue familiarity from the perspective of the defendant psychotherapist sued for sexual misconduct.

When a mental health professional is sued for malpractice, he quickly discovers that his insurer's interests are different than his own; this is particularly the case when he is sued for undue familiarity. In the landmark 1977 case of *Hartogs v. Employers Mutual Liability Insurance Co. of Wisconsin,* for example, the insurer claimed that it was not even required to provide Dr. Hartogs a legal defense, and a New York court agreed.[74] *Hartogs v. Employers Mutual* appears to be an extreme example, however, because subsequent cases have generally held that insurers are required to provide a legal defense to a malpractice suit. This is true even when allegations of criminal behavior are implicit in the claim or when a therapist has been found guilty of criminal assault in a previous trial. For example, one court held that an exclusion for criminal acts in a generic policy did not apply to a sexual misconduct claim, reasoning that the legal expenses incurred by the accused practitioner were the result of a civil malpractice and not a criminal action.[75] As a result of such decisions, the insurers affiliated with the APA and the American Psychological Association are now prepared to expend large amounts in a legal defense against a claim of undue familiarity. The APA's policy, for example, covers legal expenses up to $100,000.00.[76]

But malpractice insurers also recognize two additional factors compelling such a large amount of coverage for defense costs. First, policyholders demand that a malpractice policy provide for an adequate defense in the case of false claims, and such a high limit on defense expenditures reassures the psychotherapist who worries about a patient's manufacturing a claim of sexual misconduct, however rare such false claims may actually be.[77] Second, and not completely distinct from the first consideration, this high limit also deters potential plaintiffs from filing complaints: if a plaintiff knows that an extremely large sum will be expended in fighting her claim, she will be intimidated from filing suit, whether or not her claim has merit.

Any liability insurer will, even under ordinary circumstances, examine the plaintiff's complaint and calculate its merits, the cost of litigation, the cost of potential damages, the chance of prevailing at trial, and the alternative costs of settling. The accused practitioner's calculations, on the other hand, will be somewhat different because he must be concerned about his professional reputation and his survival as a licensed practitioner. As we shall see, since the insurance company's incentive to defend the therapist will be based on such cost-benefit calculations, much will depend on whether the policy covers or does not cover undue familiarity. And the situation is not much different if the therapist is covered by a liability insurer providing malpractice coverage under the sponsorship of the professional association to which he belongs. Although those insurers have professional peer panels to advise the company and mediate differences with accused defendants, the panel's interests are by no means the same as the defendant's, particularly if they conclude that the defendant is guilty of undue familiarity.

The sued practitioner will also discover that, in addition to his insurer, there are other stakeholders with interests different than his. If the alleged undue familiarity occurred in a medical school, hospital, or other institutional context, there will be an array of divergent interests.[78] Other stakeholders named in the suit, such as hospitals or supervisors, may sympathize with the plaintiff and wish to settle quickly and quietly to protect their institutional or personal reputations. University teaching hospitals, for example, understandably prefer to protect the university's name by settling rather than by going to court and being subject to the attendant adverse publicity. Unfortunately, it may not be in the defendant practitioner's interest to settle an undue familiarity claim if settlement means, as it increasingly does, the loss of his ability to have an affiliation with any institution or to retain his license to practice his profession.

The passage by Congress of the Health Care Quality Improvement Act (HCQIA) strengthened the mechanisms that punish unethical and incompetent physicians.[79] Among other things, the law required hospitals, medical associations, and societies to report any nontrivial sanctions imposed on physicians to state boards of medical licensure.[80] These boards are then required to enter the names of disciplined physicians in a central federal registry.[81] Most important, the act also required insurers to report any nontrivial malpractice settlement to the federal registry.[82] Hospitals now routinely access the national registry data when reviewing or awarding staff privileges. In addition, state licensing authorities, responding to the new stream of reports and motivated by consumer concerns, have become far more aggressive in the discipline of sexually exploitative physicians. Professional misconduct, implicit in a malpractice claim of undue familiarity, is therefore less likely to be concealed behind a conspiracy of silence, and it has now become almost impossible for physicians to find a safe harbor and hospital privileges in another state. In many cases, a claim of undue familiarity therefore becomes a career-ending event.

Because of the diverging and conflicting interests between him and his insurance company, the defendant practitioner accused of undue familiarity must consider the necessity of obtaining his own lawyer instead of relying on an attorney appointed by his insurer. Attorneys who are regularly paid for and supplied by insurance companies may well have a divided loyalty between the particular one-time client defendant and the insurance company that pays the bills and may well be a regular source of client referrals. Bargaining strategy for all of the parties involved will vary in different jurisdictions depending on the track record of lawyers, judges, courts, hospitals, and the penalties assessed by different state disciplinary bodies such as the state licensing authority. Although this is not the place for a full discussion of this question, clearly once the undue familiarity claim is made, every stakeholder can be expected to make self-interested calculations, including the insurance company, its agents, and the lawyers involved.

Consider the incentives for the defendant and his lawyer in a malpractice suit under a policy similar to the APA's, which excludes undue familiarity: The defendant, if he is a psychiatrist, can expect that a substantiated claim of undue familiarity will cripple or destroy his career as a licensed physician. If he loses the lawsuit, he may also be deprived of any wealth he has accumulated, because the policy does not cover damages. Nor will his policy cover a settlement, which also can be for an extremely high amount. And even if his policy does cover undue familiarity, a settlement or jury verdict against him will be reported under the HCQIA and may result in the loss of any of hospital privileges and his license to practice. Faced with such consequences, the therapist will certainly want a lawyer who will protect his interests and be his zealous advocate.

The defendant psychotherapist's interests are therefore much better served if his patient's legal complaint omits any reference to undue familiarity. Indeed, given the current climate the practitioner will be tempted to settle almost any other possible claim of negligence covered by the policy, such as misdiagnosis, failure to refer, abandonment, mismanagement of the transference not involving sexual contact, etc. It is crucial to realize that the plaintiff's lawyer may have exactly the same agenda so as to get around the caps and exclusions of the policy—caps and exclusions that limit the amount recoverable by both the victim and her lawyer, who most likely will be employed on a contingency-fee basis.

If the psychiatrist's lawyer also represents the insurance company's interests, however—as may be the case with an attorney who is supplied to the defendant by the insurer—that attorney will recognize that the insurer, who is paying his fee, benefits by the exclusionary language. He therefore will want any claim of undue familiarity to remain in the complaint in order to limit the insurer's losses. If these insurance company interests prevail, the psychiatrist loses. Whom does the lawyer serve in this dilemma?

On the one hand, both the therapist's and the patient's interests would be served by the unethical collusion of their lawyers against the insurance company as the attorneys conspire to eliminate the claim of undue familiarity. On the other hand, the doctor's lawyer may be tempted to sacrifice his mental health practitioner–client to the interests of the insurance company rather than being his zealous advocate.

For nonlawyers, worrying about these kinds of ethical problems may be unedifying, but they are certainly critical considerations for plaintiffs and defendants, as can be seen in the recent case of *Ladner v. American Home Assurance Company*.[83] In *Ladner*, a female psychologist was being sued for sexual misconduct, as well as failure to properly test, failure to follow an appropriate course of treatment, and mishandling of the transference, among other malpractice claims.[84] She had purchased a malpractice policy from American Home providing for general liability coverage of $1,000,000.00 but containing a cap of $25,000.00 for any claim involving "erotic physical contact."[85] In addition, the policy provided that, if erotic physical contact were alleged, all claims arising out of the same course of treatment would be subject to this cap.[86] Under these circumstances, the court noted,

> Counsel for [Dr. Ladner] could conceivably decide that the best defense would be to argue that, as a factual matter, the allegations of sexual misconduct were untrue, while less vigorously contesting the other types of malpractice. Such an outcome could be beneficial to [Dr. Ladner], since any damages arising out of the malpractice would in that case be subject only to the $1,000,000 limit, but for the same reason would not be beneficial to [American Home Assurance Company]. Clearly, such tactical decisions should be in the hands of an attorney whose loyalty to [Dr. Ladner] is unquestioned and not an attorney employed by [American Home] with a potential conflict of interest.[87]

As a result, the *Ladner* court ordered that American Home be enjoined from furnishing defense counsel for Dr. Ladner, and that it pay the reasonable attorneys fees of an attorney chosen by her.[88] There is no reason to believe that this scenario, openly recognized by the Ladner court, is not played out behind closed doors in many other malpractice suits involving potential claims of undue familiarity.

The Plaintiff's Lawyer and Insurance Coverage

Plaintiffs' lawyers, who generally depend on contingency fees, will of course be concerned about the caps on and exclusion of insurance coverage. Since 1992, 45 members of the American Trial Lawyers Association have shared a monthly newsletter, a major focus of which is circumventing insurance limitations for undue familiarity.[89]

One much-discussed strategy is to circumvent statutes of limitation through application of what is known as the discovery rule. Many victims of undue familiarity come forward years after the events; in fact it is not unusual to have complaints delayed by 5, 10, or even 15 years.[90] Although there is no statute of limitations for ethical complaints made to hospitals, boards of licensure, or professional associations, these statutes of limitation governing malpractice litigation require the victim to initiate the lawsuit within a designated time after the malpractice occurred. A typical statute allows the patient 3 years to file a claim.[91] However, the measurement of this limited time period can be delayed by invoking the discovery rule, which tolls or suspends the statute of limitations by allowing the time period to begin only when the "plaintiffs discover or should have discovered that they have been harmed as the result of the defendant's conduct."[92] In seeking to circumvent these limitations, plaintiffs' lawyers have argued that the discovery rule should be invoked because 1) the victims did not "discover" or "recognize" that they had been harmed because of their mental disturbance, or 2) they did not discover that the undue familiarity was the cause of their damages, or 3) the practitioner used undue influence to prevent the patient from taking legal action.[93]

These arguments in favor of the discovery rule, although not entirely convincing, are of great practical importance, because, if adopted, they grant new life to a lawsuit that previously had no hope of continuing. But many courts have rejected attempts by plaintiffs to argue that the statute of limitations should not bar their suit. In one recent case, a patient who had been raped by her psychologist claimed that the transference phenomenon prevented her from recognizing the psychological harm caused by the rape.[94] Nonetheless, a federal court ruled that the statute of limitations would not be tolled because the rape was "inherently offensive contact" of which the patient was or should have been aware at the time of the act.[95] Similarly, the Supreme Court of Tennessee recently held that a patient who was sexually abused by her therapist could not invoke the discovery rule.[96] In *Roe v. Jefferson*, the Tennessee court ruled that the patient's knowledge of and attendance at her therapist's disciplinary hearing for sexual relations with a prior client, where she was exposed to testimony that therapist-patient sex is harmful, was enough to put her on notice that a wrong had occurred.[97]

A few courts, however, have been more sympathetic. In one important earlier case, *Greenberg v. McCabe,* the court emphasized that the patient's discovery of harm was delayed by her dependence on the therapist, who assured her that his therapy was proper.[98] In *Simmons v. United States,* medical experts testified that the patient had blamed herself for the sexual contact and as a result had become depressed.[99] The court concluded that they could not decide as a matter of law that Mrs. Simmons should have known the cause of her injuries.[100] In *Riley v. Presnell,* the Massachusetts Supreme Court held that a patient who had been subject to an abhorrent therapy involving sexual relations coupled with alcohol, marijuana, and diazepam could reasonably have been unable to link the psychological injury to the therapy.[101] Plaintiffs' lawyers hope and expect that other courts will take the same approach. One should also remember that long-delayed cases such as these, if allowed under an application of the discovery rule, can be brought under the older, generic contracts in force before coverage for undue familiarity was specifically capped or excluded—as long as the defendant held an occurrence-based, generic policy for the year in which the alleged abuse took place.

The plaintiffs bar naturally wants the insurers to believe they have an arsenal of effective legal weapons. They point to decisions in which courts have found legal reasons to disregard contract language as evidence of the efficacy of malpractice suits based on sexual misconduct.[102] In addition, plaintiffs' attorneys still handle cases in which the undue familiarity began (occurred) under the old contracts. In contrast, the liability insurers convey the impression that, through the imposition of caps and exclusions, they have erected an almost impregnable defense against lawsuits involving undue familiarity. Neither side, therefore, can be expected to publish detailed information that would reveal and document the actual situation in its entirety.

However, the APA's bedpan insurer, the Psychiatrist's Purchasing Group, reported that after its exclusion of undue familiarity went into effect, they had the following experience: In the 1984–1985 fiscal year, 12.5% of claims involved and 28% of cash paid out was in satisfaction of sexual misconduct cases. In 1985–1986, the figures dropped to 5.5% of claims and 9% of cash paid out; in 1986–1987, 4.4% of claims and 7.5% of cash paid out. Since then, the rate of claims has varied from 1% to 3%.[103] These summary data, provided by Dr. Alan Levenson of the Psychiatrist's Purchasing Group, suggest that the new contractual language has successfully insulated the company against new claims of undue familiarity.[104] Furthermore, Dr. Levenson is unaware of any significant, successful strategy to mask such claims under other related claims.[105]

Nonetheless, responsible plaintiffs' lawyers continue to give assurances that their litigation strategies provide ways to circumvent the contractual language of some policies and to reach other parties, such as supervisors. Writing in *Trial*, one lawyer advised his colleagues, "Plaintiff's counsel must draft complaints with an eye to the defenses and the *coverage issues*. Counsel should take care to plead the mishandling of transference and counter-transference. *Sexual intimacy is then only an incidental outgrowth of this primary malpractice.*"[106] He also suggested that his colleagues allege breach of fiduciary relationship, outrageous conduct, and negligent infliction of emotional distress.[107] This strategy, however, would not be productive against an APA policy if the court held to the language of the contract, which excludes

... [a]ny claim, damages or cause of action based in whole or in part on actual or alleged mishandling of the transference or counter- transference phenomena, harassment, or abandonment, where the Participating member is alleged to have engaged in, or has engaged in, undue familiarity with the claimant. . . .[108]

Other plaintiffs' attorneys, however, advocate the strategy of including in the malpractice complaint concurrent claims alleging various boundary violations "other than and in addition to the sexual misconduct by the therapist."[109] For example, plaintiffs will not only allege sexual misconduct, grounding such a complaint in the mishandling of the transference, but will also seek damages for abandonment not related to the sexual misconduct, failure to refer, failure to consult, negligent prescription of medicine, failure to obtain a proper psychiatric history, failure to diagnose a dependent personality disorder, and other offenses. Jorgenson et al. point out that "the leading case in this area, *Cranford Insurance Co. v. Allwest Insurance Co.*,[110] involved an insurer that had issued a policy specifically excluding 'damages awarded in suits . . . involving undue familiarity, sexual intimacy, or assault concomitant therewith.'"[111] In that case, the court held that, although the patient's claim of mishandling of the transference was excluded since it involved sexual intimacy, the psychiatrist's abandonment of the patient was a nonexcluded risk that the insurer was required to cover.[112] The court based its rationale on its understanding that the abandonment did not involve sexual intimacy and on state law.[113] "Under California law," the court wrote, "where an insured risk and an excluded risk constitute proximate causes of an injury, a liability insurer is liable if one of the causes is covered by the policy."[114]

However, not all courts will allow plaintiffs to separate their claims in this manner. In *Chicago Insurance Co. v. Griffin,* the patient claimed that her psychologist's mismanagement of the transference was separate from the sexual conduct, and therefore her claims extended beyond the policy exclusion for sexual activity.[115] In rejecting this contention, the court held that the sexual misconduct was the "essential element" of the claim and could not be so separated; the malpractice claims were therefore excluded from coverage.[116] And a federal court found sex to be such an essential element even when the patient's attorneys had refrained from mentioning sexual misconduct altogether: In *Govar v. Chicago Insurance,*[117] the court held that a malpractice claim alleging only that the therapist failed to exercise the proper amount of degree and skill was in fact a claim entirely centered on sexual misconduct.[118] These decisions indicate that, if sex is an "essential element"[119] of the plaintiff's claim, attempts to plead concurrent proximate causes or to exclude sexual misconduct entirely from the complaint may fail.

All of this legal maneuvering confirms our impression that the victim-plaintiff, as well as the practitioner-defendant, will want to downplay or omit including sexual intimacy in the complaint. Unfortunately, there is no definitive evidence about the frequency of such camouflaged litigation. Cases purportedly involving hidden instances of sexual misconduct naturally focus on nonsexual boundary violations and other forms of misconduct. Furthermore, most of the reported cases in which plaintiffs have successfully litigated sexual misconduct claims involve insurance companies that capped or did not specifically exclude undue familiarity.

Punitive Damages

It is important to realize that the critical factor in all of these strategic decisions is the money that a court can award to the victim of sexual misconduct—that is, the "damages." The legal term *damages* encompasses two different theoretical justifications and purposes: compensatory damages and punitive damages. As the name suggests, compensatory damages are awarded to recompense the victim for the actual damage or losses resulting from the mental health professional's negligence or sexual misconduct.[120] The purpose of such damages is therefore, in the language of the law, "to make the party whole"—that is, to restore the abused patient to the place she would have occupied had the sexual misconduct not occurred, to the extent that it is possible to measure the patient's injury in monetary terms.[121] In contrast, punitive damages—also known as "exemplary damages"—exist to punish the physician and to deter him or others like him "from similar extreme misconduct in the future."[122] Unlike compensatory damages, punitive damages are not limited to the loss suffered by the patient, and therefore often can be much *larger* than the amount awarded as compensatory damages. In cases under the earlier generation of standard or generic policies, the question naturally arose whether the insurance companies were required to cover punitive damages as well as compensatory damages. In one of the first malpractice cases in which a male psychiatrist sexually abused his female patient, *Roy v. Hartogs,* the trial court originally awarded compensatory damages of $50,000.00 while allowing punitive damages of over $100,000.00.[123] The award was eventually limited on appeal, wherein the court held that the evidence did not justify the awarding of any punitive damages and that the compensatory damages were to be limited to a maximum of $25,000.00.[124] Subsequent courts have given larger awards and have allowed punitive damages. For example, a decade later, in the notorious case of *Mazza v. Medical Mutual Life Insurance Co. of North Carolina,* the jury awarded compensatory damages of $102,000.00 and punitive damages of over $500,000.00 on grounds that the psychiatrist had become involved in an affair with the patient's wife.[125] The compensatory and punitive damages were upheld on appeal.[126]

However, courts have not uniformly determined that punitive damages should be covered by professional liability insurance. For example, in one case involving a dentist accused of sexual molestation, *Public Service Mutual Insurance Company v. Goldfarb,* the New York Court of Appeals determined that an insurer would not, as a matter of public policy, be liable to indemnify the dentist in the event that a trial

court awarded punitive damages to his patient.[127] Such punitive damages, the *Goldfarb* court reasoned, are only to be awarded as the result
of intentional, not negligent, conduct, and therefore, allowing them
would violate New York's public policy against indemnifying such intentional acts.[128] The implications for mental health professionals involved in similar litigation are substantial: even if they have insurance
coverage under their policy, it may not protect against a monumental
punitive damages award.

The problem of damages, therefore, is intimately related to all of the
concerns previously discussed in this chapter. As we have seen, the
monumental punitive and compensatory damages awards have driven
the insurance companies to cap or exclude claims of sexual misconduct—and these caps or exclusions are generally upheld. It is therefore
only in the context of the older-generation generic policies that the issue of insurance coverage of punitive damages for sexual misconduct
arises. Insurers that have issued those policies on an occurrence basis
may still be liable for these extremely large punitive damages awards in
some jurisdictions. The application of the discovery rule further increases the risk to the insurers. However, since most policies now contain caps or exclusions on undue familiarity claims,[129] victims of sexual
misconduct will increasingly find that the insurers' deep pocket is
closed—unless, of course, their attorneys can develop a strategy that
will circumvent the contractual language.

Conclusion

At present it seems that insurers are continuing to find new ways to
avoid indemnifying psychotherapists accused of sexual misconduct.
The policies issued by the bedpan insurers for the APA and the American Psychological Association, for example, now exclude all claims of
sexual misconduct while at the same time providing for expensive defenses. Recent court decisions, however, demonstrate that plaintiffs' attorneys continue to seek strategies to circumvent the insurers with
varying degrees of success. But all of these strategies, which have been
devised by both sides in response to technical legal opinions, obscure
the fundamental moral question: Who can and should reimburse the
innocent victim of sexual misconduct? The answer to that question de-

pends on how one conceives of both medical malpractice insurance and the psychopathology of psychotherapists who sexually victimize their patients.

Although there is an extensive literature discussed elsewhere in this volume on the psychopathology of the offending psychotherapists, these psychodynamic and diagnostic formulations unfortunately offer no clear guidance on the policy question of insurance coverage. One might argue on clinical grounds that a psychotherapist with an exploitative, narcissistic personality disorder should not be protected by insurance and that a psychotherapist with a transient depression should be: the depressed psychiatrist is psychologically impaired in a manner that the narcissistic therapist is not. The depressed practitioner, in this view, is not as venal as the antisocial one. Although such considerations might be quite relevant to a medical disciplinary board, if both psychotherapists have victimized their patients, each patient would seem to be equally deserving of compensation. There is nonetheless an important moral intuition in this diagnostic distinction. We believe that the narcissistic or the antisocial psychotherapist is exploiting his role as psychotherapist in a way that the depressed psychotherapist is not. This kind of distinction is certainly familiar to psychotherapists, but it tends to be overshadowed by the moral impulse to condemn the exploitative conduct whatever its motivation. The same moral concerns, moreover, make it difficult if not impossible to focus, in each case of sexual misconduct, on the interpersonal dynamic between the particular patient and offending psychotherapist to decide whether or not that practitioner should be indemnified and, therefore, whether that particular patient should be compensated for her victimization.

We therefore intend neither to blame the victim nor excuse the psychotherapist when we suggest that undue familiarity could, for the narrow purpose of determining insurance liability, be considered akin to an occupational hazard. Not every member of a particular occupation succumbs to its inherent hazard. For example, we know that although physicians and nurses are at greater risk of addiction to prescription drugs because they have access to them, not all are addicted. But enough do succumb to put significant numbers of patients at risk. Although such behavior by physicians and nurses cannot be excused, it can be anticipated. Such addiction becomes an occupational risk, the effects of which an insurer might be expected to cover despite the moral inclination to condemn the addicted practitioner. The concept of occupational hazard neither minimizes nor justifies addiction. In the very same sense, undue familiarity might be considered an occupational hazard for psychotherapists. In *Love*, the Supreme Court of Minnesota seems to have been following this line of reasoning: they condemned the psychotherapist's sexual misconduct as "aberrant and unacceptable" but concluded that the risk of such behavior, due to the presence of the transference phenomenon, was inherent in the occupation and therefore should be covered.[130]

In addition, viewing sexual misconduct by psychotherapists as an occupational risk allows for public policy arguments favoring compensation of the psychotherapists' victims, arguments that depend on a particular conception of the nature of malpractice insurance. If malpractice insurance is thought to be, at its fundamental level, merely a contract into which the parties enter freely, then a marketplace philosophy honoring such freedom to contract demands that caps and exclusions on sexual misconduct claims be upheld. Such caps and exclusions are, after all, part of the contract to which both the insurer and the insured practitioner have agreed. This view has been the position of many courts that have considered this question, even those that might be considered sympathetic to the victim of sexual misconduct.[131] However, there are a few court decisions that suggest a more radical view, although none adopts that view entirely. These courts conceptualize medical malpractice insurance as a victim compensation fund designed not only to protect the expectations of the parties to the contract (i.e., the psychotherapist and the insurance company) but also to protect the innocent third party: the patient, usually a woman, who has been harmed and who has been awarded damages in a court of law.[132] If malpractice insurance is to be so conceived, then a plausible argument can be made that public policy should disallow insurers from limiting their exposure to this type of "occupational risk." Much as the public policy of some states requires automobile insurers to provide a certain minimum level of coverage, so the argument goes, public policy requires a minimum level of coverage for the victims of undue familiarity—the victims of a risk that is inherent in the profession. As of this date, however, no court has taken the radical approach of stating that such minimum levels are required by public policy, and in fact several have expressly declined to do so.[133] But the idea of medical malpractice insurance being at least partly a victim compensation fund has been introduced. Only time will tell if courts will take the next steps and view this partial purpose to be compelling enough to demand coverage, or even view insurance exclusively as such a fund.

We do not suggest that this approach will resolve all of the competing considerations. As we have indicated, the cost of liability insurance would escalate, the market would be disrupted, and some bedpan insurers might go bankrupt. Perhaps the solution, if there is one, lies in the direction that the courts traditionally look when determining public policy: the state legislature.[134] Courts that have considered plaintiffs' public policy challenges to caps and exclusions, and insurers' public policy objections to indemnifying undue familiarity, invariably look first to state law to determine legislative intent.[135] Therefore, until state legislatures write clear state laws favoring the compensation of victims of sexual misconduct by psychotherapists, such compensation will be unlikely, given the primacy of contract in American jurisprudence. At least one state has already passed a law mandating a minimum level of coverage for health care professionals,[136] and some states provide for civil causes of action for patients who have been sexually abused by their psychotherapists.[137] Roughly one-fifth have passed criminal statutes penalizing such misconduct.[138] It therefore is not entirely fanciful to suggest that other laws might be written to favor victim compensation through insurance. In effect, the state would force practitioners to pay the higher premiums necessary to cover the victims of undue familiarity under even a minimal policy. Given the financial and political realities of the mid-1990s, however, it is entirely possible that state legislatures will view such laws as another unwanted expansion of governmental regulation.

Without resolution of these conflicts by statute or regulation, insurers can be expected to adopt the exclusionary language in the APA's contract; and in response, plaintiffs' attorneys will have to devise new legal strategies. The struggle will continue,[139] because there are in fact good social policy grounds on both sides: economic viability and victim compensation. This dilemma confronts the legal system in many areas where money and morality collide.

Appendix 3-1. Case Illustrations

The following cases provide useful illustrations of the problematic issues inherent in insuring against sexual misconduct. A brief review should familiarize the psychotherapist possessing little or no legal background with the relevant issues. The cases are listed and discussed in chronological order. (Cases focusing on statute of limitations or discovery questions have been omitted. This compilation is not intended to be exhaustive.)

Zipkin v. Freeman, 436 SW2d 753 (1969). The Missouri Supreme Court holds that standard policy language covering "professional services rendered or which should have been rendered" includes a psychiatrist's mismanagement of the transference phenomenon resulting in various boundary violations, including inducing patient to leave husband, to invest in farm for psychiatrist, and to move into apartment above psychiatrist's office.

Hartogs v. Employers Mutual Liability Insurance Co. of Wisconsin, 391 NYS2d 962 (AppDiv 1977). New York court holds that public policy against indemnifying immoral conduct prevents a psychiatrist from recovering his legal costs because he knew that his sexually based treatment existed not as part of the doctor-patient relationship but merely to "accomplish his personal satisfaction." 391 NYS at 964. However, court states that liability policy does not exist solely for protection of the insured, but that the injured person is to be protected as well. 391 NYS at 964. Distinguishes relationship of victim and insurer from insured physician and insurer, suggesting that victim may sustain an action versus insurer even though the insured psychiatrist may not. 391 NYS at 964–965.

Pacific Mutual Insurance Co. v. Goldfarb, 425 NE2d 810 (NY 1981). Malpractice insurer is obligated to defend a malpractice suit for sexual misconduct arising in the course of dental treatment, as policy clearly indicated the intent to defend against and indemnify damages arising out of unlawful or inappropriate physical contact occurring during treatment. 425 NE2d at 813. Punitive damages not allowed, as such damages would violate New York State's public policy against indemnifying intentional acts, but coverage for compensatory damages would be allowed if the dentist had not intended to cause injury by his sexual misconduct even though the misconduct itself was intentional. Id.

Vigilant Insurance Co. v. Kambly, 319 NW2d 382 (Mich App 1982). Public policy against insuring of criminal or intentional acts is *not* applicable to psychiatrist who induced patient to engage in sexual relations with him as a part of her psychotherapy. 319 NW2d at 384–385. Dispositive factors are 1) the lack of probability that the psychiatrist was induced to engage in the unlawful conduct by reliance on insurance coverage; 2) the small chance that allowing coverage would induce similar misconduct in the future; 3) the absence of evidence that the policy was obtained in contemplation of a violation of the law; and 4) the great public interest in protecting the interest of the injured party through compensation. 319 NW2d at 385 (citations omitted).

St. Paul Fire and Marine Insurance Co. v. Mitchell, 296 SE2d 126 (Ga App 1982). Psychiatrist's mishandling of the transference phenomenon that resulted in sex with his patient was within his generic policy's standard provisions providing for defense of claims "arising out of the performance of professional services." 296 SE2d at 127. Distinguished from *Hartogs,* supra, in that psychiatrist in this case had not been found to be a wrongdoer and therefore insurer was obligated to defend him. 296 SE2d at 128.

L.L. v. Medical Protective Co., 362 NW2d 174 (Wisc App 1984). **Review denied,** 367 NW2d 223 (Wisc 1985). Because sexual misconduct derives from a mismanagement of the transference phenomenon, psychiatrist's sexual contact (fellatio) with his patient is within the language of his generic malpractice policy covering claims for damages "based on professional services rendered or which should have been rendered." 362 NW at 175. Court states that Wisconsin public policy views a liability insurance contract as existing for the benefit of injured members of the public; therefore, a malpractice insurance policy that was intended to benefit such members was not in violation of public policy. 362 NW at 179.

Mazza v. Medical Mutual Insurance Co. of North Carolina, 319 SE2d 217 (NC 1984). In matter of a psychiatrist who seduced his patient's wife, the North Carolina Supreme Court holds that public policy does not preclude coverage for $500,000 punitive damages award, and that the language in the policy covering "claims . . . arising out of the performance of professional services" was broad enough to cover such action. 319 SE2d at 219. The court states that recent trend of courts in considering public policy objections has been to allow coverage for punitive damages, even in cases of willful and wanton negligence as opposed to intentional torts. 319 SE2d at 219–220.

Frankenmuth Mutual Insurance Co. v. Kompus, 354 NW2d 303 (Mich App 1984). This appeal does not involve professional liability insurance; the court was asked to interpret coverage of a homeowner's policy issued to a psychiatrist who engaged in homosexual activities with patient under the guise of providing therapy, and who was subsequently convicted of third-degree criminal sexual conduct. 354 NW2d at 306. (The malpractice insurers were previously held to have duty to defend psychiatrist. 354 NW2d at 306.) Homeowner insurers have no duty to defend against sexual misconduct claim because of a "business pursuits" exclusion in their policies, such exclusions being determined by a two-pronged test of continuity and profit motive. 354 NW2d at 306–308. In addition, homeowner's coverage for injuries caused by an "occurrence" does not cover injuries resulting from sexual misconduct, because the occurrence is defined by the policies as an "accident" and the psychiatrist's actions were intentional, not an accident. 354 NW2d at 309–310.

Smith v. St. Paul Fire and Marine Insurance Co., 353 NW2d 130 (Minn 1984). Medical doctor (not a psychiatrist) sexually molested boys under his care and eventually pleaded guilty to criminal sexual assault in the fourth degree. Court looks to the "plain meaning" of the generic policy's language and finds that the policy contemplated incorrect or improper medical treatment only, and that sexual misconduct involved neither the providing nor the withholding of professional services. 353 NW2d at 132.

Hirst v. St. Paul Fire and Marine Insurance Co., 683 P2d 440, 444 (Idaho CtApp 1984). Insurer not liable to indemnify a nonpsychiatric physician who drugged and sexually assaulted a young patient during an examination of a hand injury, as such an assault does not constitute the "professional services" that the physician's generic policy covered. Intentional sexual assault does not constitute professional services under the policy provisions as, although the patient had been drugged by the physician, the court finds no causal connection between the administration of the drugs and the harm claimed by the patient. 683 P2d at 444.

Standlee v. St. Paul Fire and Marine Insurance Co., 693 P2d 1101 (Idaho App 1984). Same physician as in *Hirst*, supra, but different victim. Professional liability policy issued to physician did not cover a sexual assault committed in a hospital, because the malpractice policy was of the generic type related to professional services. 693 P2d at 1102. In addition, the physician's office liability policy did not cover liability for sexual molestation, as coverage was limited to damages arising from a personal injury caused by an "accidental event." 693 P2d at 1102. The clause requiring coverage for "losses the physician is legally responsible for that result from actions necessary to his work" did not create an ambiguity requiring indemnity for all intentional acts. 693 P2d at 1102–1103.

Gilbreath v. St. Paul Fire and Marine Insurance Co., 685 P2d 729 (Ariz 1984). In case of sexually abused child, court upholds policy exclusion for any injury to those in care, custody or control of insured day care center. 685 P2d at 733.

Vigilant Insurance Co. v. Employers Insurance of Wausau, 626 F Supp 262 (SDNY 1986). Psychiatrist engaged in nude "primal therapy" sessions and sexual intercourse with one patient and ordered another to disrobe in his apartment. The court holds that the generic policy language can be construed to include sexual misconduct due to the presence in therapy of the transference phenomenon, which renders the patient especially vulnerable. 626 F Supp at 265–266. Public policy objections to insuring against intentional acts not applicable due to evidence that the physician did not intend to harm his patients based on testimony regarding his statements of concern for them. 626 F Supp at 267.

Sphere Insurance Co., Ltd., v. Rosen, 1986 WL 5721 (EDPa). Court upholds sexual misconduct exclusion in malpractice policy held by psychiatrist who developed "direct therapy." 1986 WL 5721 *2. No duty to defend Dr. Rosen since insurer was not bound to indemnify him, a result which goes back to *Hartogs,* supra. Id.

Cranford Insurance Co., Inc., v. Allwest Insurance Co., 645 F Supp 1440 (NDCal 1986). Exclusion for sexual misconduct in malpractice policy upheld in case of psychiatrist who entered into sexual relationship with patient shortly before terminating therapy. Victim allowed to claim negligent acts in addition to and separate from the claim of undue familiarity. 645 F Supp at 1444. The court finds the psychiatrist's abandonment to be a possible cause, in and of itself, of victim's injuries. 645 F Supp at 1444. Jorgenson et al. point out that the court here finds that the sexual abuse and the abandonment were concurrent proximate causes of the patient's psychological injuries.[140]

St. Paul Fire and Marine Insurance Co. v. Asbury, 720 P2d 540 (Ariz App 1986). Court finds that sexual abuse by gynecologist is covered by a generic malpractice policy, agreeing with the trial court that the tortious conduct occurred during the treatment of patients and was inseparable from the act of providing professional services. 720 P2d at 542. (Gynecologist had performed "improper manipulations" while performing examinations. 720 P2d at 541.) Citing *Kambly* factors, supra, court finds no public policy objection to coverage. 720 P2d at 542. States that "the public policy of Arizona favors protecting the interests of injured parties." Id.

Washington Insurance Guaranty Association v. Hicks, 744 P2d 625 (Wash App 1987).   Chiropractor's generic malpractice policy does not cover his engaging in sexual intercourse with a patient during a treatment session at office. Although the insurer of a therapist should reasonably expect that the transference phenomenon is central to therapy, an insurer of a chiropractor should not be held to the same assumption. 744 P2d at 627.

S.C. Medical Malpractice Liability Insurance JUA v. Ferry, 354 SE2d 378 (SC 1987).   Oral surgeon's generic malpractice policy does not cover original allegation of sexual misconduct, as such misconduct is not a professional service, but an intentional tort. 354 SE2d at 381. However, the insurer has a duty to defend amended complaints that add claims of negligence and recklessness, alleging failure to exercise ordinary care in administering anesthesia or medication, failure to perform physical examination before surgery, failure to obtain informed consent and to properly record doses of medications. 354 SE2d at 380-81.

St. Paul Fire and Marine Insurance Co. v. Ouintana, 419 NW2d 60 (Mich App 1988).   Generic policy does not cover damages arising from sexual assault by an EEG technician because the misconduct did not lie within the term "professional services"—a term contemplating "improper or incorrect administration of the EEG, not the sexual assault. . . . " 419 NW2d at 63.

Snyder v. National Union Fire Insurance Co., 688 F Supp 932 (SDNY 1988).   Despite criminal act exclusion, insurer must defend plastic surgeon convicted of raping patient because the patient's civil complaint alleged acts of medical malpractice separate and apart from the sexual abuse—including negligence, wrongful drug injection, failure to obtain informed consent, and intentional infliction of emotional distress—which fall within the generic policy's coverage for "a medical incident." 688 F Supp at 933–938.

Govar v. Chicago Insurance Co., 879 F2d 1581 (8th Cir 1989).   Victim of undue familiarity amended complaint to delete all references to sexual misconduct by psychologist. Court finds that policy exclusion for sexual misconduct nevertheless applies, as entire case centers on sexual misconduct which "was so entertwined with . . . malpractice as to be inseparable." 879 F2d at 1583.

Standard Fire and Insurance Co. v. Blakeslee, 771 **P2d 1172 (Wash App 1989).** Dentist sexually assaults sedated patient. Court holds that generic malpractice policy provides no coverage for damages when "the physician's sexual contact with his patient is not necessitated by the particular course of medical treatment." 771 P2d at 1176 (citing *Hicks,* supra, at 625). States that "[i]n sexual abuse cases, our Supreme Court has held that an intent to injure is presumed as a matter of law" and therefore upholds an exclusion for intentional injuries in a general liability policy issued by insurer. 771 P2d at 1174.

Horace Mann Insurance Co. v. Analisa N., **214 Cal App 3d 850 (1989).** Insurer not liable for judgment rendered against a third-grade teacher for sexually abusing one of his students during lunch breaks and after school. Policy "requires, at the very least, that an insured event occur while the teacher is engaged in an activity which is reasonably related to the goal of educating children." Court sympathetic to victim but says sympathy "does not give us the power to expand the risks . . . [insurer] assumed in issuing a policy. . . . Indeed were we to do so we would only increase the cost and availability [sic] of insurance for those teachers who run no small risk of liability by engaging in a myriad of extracurricular activities designed to enrich our children's lives." 214 Cal App 3d at 856.

St. Paul Fire and Marine Insurance Co. v. Love, **447 NW2d 5 (Minn CtApp 1989). Affirmed by 459 NW2d 698 (Minn 1990).** The Minnesota Court of Appeals holds that a generic malpractice policy covers sexual misconduct by a psychologist due to the existence of the transference phenomenon in the therapeutic milieu, and the court's determination is that such mishandling and not the sexual conduct itself is the proximate cause of the plaintiff's injuries. 447 NW2d at 10–11.

Govar v. Chicago Insurance Co., **879 F2d 1581 (8th Cir 1989).** Patient filed a medical malpractice suit against her psychologist, who had engaged her in sexual activity. Patient obtained a judgment and brought a declaratory judgment action against psychologist's malpractice insurer, seeking a declaration that insurer was required to pay the judgment against psychologist. Applying Arkansas law, the appellate court agreed with the district court that the malpractice policy excluded coverage based on a clause excluding coverage for claims arising out of sexual acts. The court held that the patient's entire case was centered on sex and that the sexual relationship between the patient and the psychologist was "so intertwined with the psychologist's malpractice as to be inseparable." 879 F2d at 1582.

Love v. St. Paul Fire and Marine Insurance Co., 459 NW2d 698 (Minn 1990). Affirming *St. Paul Fire and Marine Insurance Co. v. Love,* supra, the Supreme Court of Minnesota holds that when the transference phenomenon pervades the therapeutic alliance, generic insurance policy will cover sexual misconduct because the insurer agrees to provide coverage for risks inherent in psychotherapy. The psychotherapist must encourage some aspects of transference and discourage others: "This may be difficult to do and presents an occupational risk." 459 NW at 702.

St. Paul Fire and Marine Insurance Co. v. Vigilant Insurance Co., 919 F2d 235 (4th Cir 1990). Psychiatrist hugs and kisses patient during office visits, then engages in sexual intercourse with patient after terminating therapy and after policy expires. 919 F2d at 238. Court holds that insurer must defend because patient's complaint seeks relief not just for the time sexual actions commenced but for actions occurring during the entire doctor-patient relationship as a whole, which would encompass the policy period. 919 F2d at 240.

St. Paul Fire and Marine Insurance Co. v. D.H.L., 459 NW2d 704 (Minn 1990). Narrowing *Love v. St. Paul Fire and Marine Insurance Co.*, 459 NW 698 (Minn 1990), supra, Minnesota Supreme Court reverses and remands appeals court finding in favor of coverage. Holds that transference will not be automatically presumed just because the professional being sued is a mental health professional, but must be developed through expert testimony. 459 NW2d at 706.

St. Paul Insurance Co. of Illinois v. Cromeans, 771 F Supp 349 (NDAla 1991). Insurer who had issued generic policy not required to defend or indemnify a physician who filmed two naked juvenile patients, masturbated in front of them, and fondled them. Finds such sexual misconduct to be intentional, which the insuring against would violate public policy.

Niedzielski v. St. Paul Fire and Marine Insurance Co., 589 A2d 130 (NH 1991). Dentist's generic policy provides no coverage for sexual assault on patient, as such assault does not constitute the "professional services" within policy's meaning. Distinguishes situation of dentist from that of psychotherapist who exploits the intimate doctor-patient relationship to obtain sex. 589 A2d at 132.

Rivera v. Medical Liability Insurance Co., 814 P2d 71 (Nev 1991). Gynecologist convicted of forcibly raping patient. Court upholds malpractice policy's exclusion for acts intended to cause injury or damages, because rape is "an act which the assailant knows with substantial certainty will cause harm. . . ." 814 P2d at 73–74. Also upholds intentional, criminal, and sexual acts exclusions under public policy considerations due to difficulty of determining acts that physician committed only because he was insured, due to traditional contract considerations upholding insurer's ability to set terms of policy, and due to expectations of purchasers. 814 P2d at 74.

St. Paul Fire and Marine Insurance Co. v. Mori, 486 NW2d 803 (Minn App 1992). Further narrows the Minnesota Supreme Court's decision in *Love*, supra. "The presence of some transference is insufficient to constitute the providing or withholding of professional services. There must be a conscious decision by the therapist to attempt to induce transference before the mishandling of the transference phenomenon will come within the holding of *Love*." 486 NW2d at 809. Finds no evidence that a gynecologist intended to enter into a therapeutic alliance with his patient that was designed to induce love-transference. Id.

Roe v. Federal Insurance Co., 587 NE2d 214 (Mass 1992). Court finds no coverage for damages under standard policy for dentist who allegedly sexually molested his patient. States that there must be medical or dental act or service that harms the patient and not an act that requires no professional skill. 587 NE2d at 217. Case distinguished from situation of therapist and patient operating within the transference phenomenon. 587 NE2d at 218.

Snyder v. Major, 789 F Supp 646 (SDNY 1992). On reargument 818 F Supp 68 (SDNY 1993). Same case as *Snyder v. National Union Fire Insurance Co.*, supra, in which a plastic surgeon raped a sedated patient. Adheres to the majority view that "sexual conduct is not a medical incident for insurance purposes unless the physician is a psychiatrist and the sexual incident arises out of a therapeutic relationship." 789 F Supp at 651.

St. Paul Fire and Marine Insurance Co. v. Shernow, 610 A2d 1281 (1992). Dentist's intentional sexual assault on sedated patient was so "inextricably intertwined and inseparable" from negligent administration of nitrous oxide causing permanent injury that insurer must extend coverage under a generic policy. 610 A2d at 1285. No public policy objection to coverage, as no finding of intent to injure patient. 610 A2d at 1284–1285.

Collins v. Covenant Mutual Insurance Co., 604 NE2d 1190 (Ind App 2 Dist 1992). Sexual misconduct claim not within generic policy coverage of nonpsychiatric physician who engaged in sexual relationship with patient, impregnated her, surreptitiously aborted fetus, mistreated patient, and failed to treat wound inflicted on her. 604 NE2d at 1195–1197. Distinguishes situation from a therapist-patient relationship "in which the risk of mishandling the transference phenomenon is an occupational hazard generally within the scope of professional liability coverage." 604 NE2d at 1196–1197.

Vetter v. St. Paul Fire and Marine Insurance Co., 844 F Supp 1352 (D Minn 1992), affirmed 12 F3d 105 (8th Cir, 1993). In an action arising out of professional malpractice, patient entered into an agreement with psychotherapist whereby the psychotherapist admitted liability and damages and the patient agreed to seek recourse only against the insurer. The court concluded that 1) the settlement was reasonable and prudent; 2) the psychotherapist did not violate duty to cooperate with insurer by entering into the agreement; and 3) the alleged mishandling of the transference phenomenon and countertransference by engaging in sexual relationship with patient constituted professional malpractice and was covered by the policy. 844 F Supp at 1355–1356.

St. Paul Fire and Marine Insurance Co. v. Downs, 617 NE2d 338 (Ill App 1 Dist 1993). Upholds trial court opinion granting summary judgment to insurer of mental health center on technical grounds of collateral estoppel, but also states that, as matter of law, a psychotherapist who engages in sexual misconduct with a patient cannot be said to operate outside of his employment, and therefore the therapist's employer may be liable for such misconduct under the theory of respondeat superior. 617 NE2d at 344–345.

New Mexico Physicians Mutual Liability Co. v. LaMure, 860 P2d 734 (NM 1993). Physician convicted of sexual assault of a minor, criminal sexual penetration, and extortion. Court finds no coverage under generic policy, as sexual misconduct is not a covered professional service. 860 P2d at 738. Also upholds policy exclusion for criminal actions on both contractual and public policy grounds. 860 P2d at 740.

Stephen G. by Robert G. v. Herget, 505 NW2d 422 (Wisc App 1993). Review denied. 510 NW2d 136 (Wis 1993). Court rejects idea that transference occurred between a dentist and his patient and determines that sexual assault by dentist upon sedated patient did not arise out of the rendering of or failure to render professional services as required for coverage in generic malpractice policy. 505 NW2d at 424. Distinguishes case from *Shernow*, supra, which involved serious physical injury to victim caused by negligent administration of nitrous oxide. 505 NW2d at 427.

Lindeheimer v. St. Paul Fire and Marine Insurance Co., 643 So2d 636 (Fla App 3 Dist 1994). **Affirmed and remanded.** 67 F3d 305 (9th Cir 1995).   Court holds that insurer who had issued a professional liability insurance policy does not cover acts of sexual misconduct, because the dentist's sexual assault was not causally connected to the provision of professional services. 643 So2d at 638.

American Home Assurance Co. v. Cohen, 815 F Supp 365 (WD Wash 1993).   Due to presence in malpractice policy of both cap on claims of sexual misconduct and exclusion for wrongful acts, policy is ambiguous and therefore construed to provide coverage for psychologist who engaged in intercourse with a patient. 815 F Supp at 369. Provision limiting all claims, including nonsexual ones, to sublimit of $25,000 once undue familiarity is alleged "at any time, either in a complaint, during discovery, at trial or otherwise . . . " violates public policy by discouraging disclosure of and compensation for harms caused by sexual misconduct and by focusing on the innocent victim to deny coverage. 815 F Supp at 371. Rejects argument that policy unfairly discriminates against women, finding instead that policy is gender neutral and limitation is valid due to increased risk posed to insurer by sexual misconduct claims. 815 F Supp at 372–373.

Chicago Insurance Co. v. Griffin, 817 F Supp 861 (D Hawaii 1993).   Rejects argument by victim of undue familiarity that psychologist's mismanagement of transference phenomenon is separate from sexual misconduct claims. Relying on *Govar,* supra, and *Cranford,* supra, court finds that sexual misconduct is an essential element of patient's malpractice claim and therefore invokes policy exclusion for sexual misconduct. 817 F Supp at 867.

Dillion v. Callaway, 609 NE2d 424 (Ind CtApp 1993).   Court holds that injuries resulting from sexual relationship that occurred during therapy sessions were covered under the Medical Malpractice Act, despite alleged public policy against insuring intentional acts. 609 NE2d at 428.

Ladner v. American Home Assurance Co., 607 NYS2d 296 (AD 1 Dept 1994).   Court finds a potential for conflict of interest between psychologist and her insurer, who had issued a capped policy containing sublimit of $25,000 for claims involving erotic physical contact and all other claims growing out of the same or related course of treatment.

American Home Assurance Co. v. Stone, **864 F Supp 767 (ND Ill 1994) Affirmed. 61 F3d 1321 (7th Cir 1995) as modified (Aug 24, 1995).** Case of psychotherapist/divorce mediator who seduced patient; psychotherapist's malpractice policy limited to $25,000 claims of sexual misconduct and all related claims growing out of the same or related course of treatment. Court rejects argument that upholding limitation would unfairly force a "blameless" employer to be accountable for sexual misconduct of employee, would be contrary to reasonable expectations of third-party beneficiaries, and would violate public policy of encouraging settlements. 864 F Supp 777. Provision also held not to violate public policy against sex discrimination despite disproportionate impact on women, and not to violate public policy of encouraging reporting sexual misconduct. Id at 774. Finds limitation unambiguous. Id at 773.

American Home Assurance Co. v. Cohen, **881 P2d 1001 (Wash 1994).** Certification from the U.S. Court of Appeals for the Ninth Circuit in case of psychologist sued for nine separate claims of malpractice, including sexual misconduct, failure to treat, abandonment, etc. 881 P2d at 1003. Malpractice policy provision limited coverage for claims of sexual misconduct to $25,000, as well as all claims arising out of the same or related course of treatment, whether involving sexual misconduct or not. 881 P2d at 1003. Washington Supreme Court finds limitation does not offend the public good because it is not in conflict with any public policy mandating full compensation or insurance coverage and is related to an identifiable risk to the insurer. 881 P2d at 1008. But expansion of limitation to cover claims of nonsexual malpractice violates public policy in that it discourages victims from reporting sexual misconduct "so that other clients will be protected from unethical, unprofessional and harmful conduct of offending psychologists." 881 P2d at 1010.

P.S. v. Psychiatric Coverage, Ltd., **887 SW2d 622 (Mo App 1994).** Patient and her husband brought medical malpractice action against psychologist and psychologist's employer. The court held that employer was not liable under respondeat superior for damages resulting from psychologist's sexual relations with patient, because psychologist was not acting within scope and course of his employment as therapist in having sexual relations with patient. 887 SW2d at 624-625.

St. Paul Fire and Marine Insurance Co. v. F.H., 55 F3d 1420 (9th Cir 1995). The court held that under Alaska law, professional liability insurance policy's exclusion of coverage for criminal acts by volunteers in big brother/big sister program did not apply to sexual abuse by program's executive director. The executive director's acts were covered by the insurance policy because he placed the victim with himself and acted as a big brother, an act which was within the scope of his employment and caused the ultimate abuse. 55 F3d at 1422–1425.

Doe v. Madison Center Hospital, 652 NE2d 101 (Ind App 1995). Minor psychiatric patient and mother brought action against mental health care facility and mental health counselor for assault, battery, and intentional infliction of emotional distress, alleging that counselor coerced sexual intercourse with patient, resulting in her contracting venereal diseases. The court held that plaintiff's allegations did not fall within the purview of the Indiana Medical Malpractice Act, because the complaint did not contend that there was a therapist-patient relationship between the counselor and the patient. "The alleged acts, although occurring during Jane Doe's confinement in the Hospital for psychiatric care and treatment, were not designed to promote her health. Neither do they call into question King's use of skill or expertise as a health care provider." 652 NE2d at 104–107.

McConaghy v. RLI Insurance Co., 882 F Supp 540 (ED Va 1995). Marital counselor engaged in a romantic and sexual relationship with patient while continuing to counsel him and his wife. The couple subsequently divorced and brought suit against the counselor for negligence, breach of fiduciary duty, and intentional infliction of emotional distress, alleging nonsexual acts of malpractice in addition to the sexually related acts. The defendant's malpractice insurer argued that the relevant policy's $50,000 sublimit on claims involving sexual misconduct created a cap for the entire suit, even though nonsexual malpractice was also alleged. (The policy as a whole had a $500,000 limit.) The plaintiffs challenged on public policy grounds, arguing that such a limit would discourage injured parties from reporting sexual misconduct, while possibly encouraging mental health professionals to engage in sexual misconduct in order to limit their liability for nonsexual malpractice. Although acknowledging that it was "deeply troubled" by the apparent inequity of the policy sublimit, the court nonetheless upheld the policy provision, stating that there was no "clear indication" from the state legislature or supreme court of contrary public policy warranting disruption of the contract term.

Block v. Gomez, 549 NW2d 783 (Wis App 1996).   A patient who had a sexual relationship with her drug abuse counselor brought action against her counselor and his clinic employer. The court held that 1) the transference phenomenon did not make the drug abuse counselor's sexual relationship with the patient inseparable from his therapeutic relationship with patient for purposes of the clinic's vicarious liability, and 2) the clinic was not vicariously liable under the doctrine of respondeat superior for the counselor's actions, because the counselor undisputedly stepped aside from the clinic's business to procure a purely personal benefit: a sexual relationship with Block. 549 NW2d at 788.

Legion Insurance Co. v. Vemuri, WL 757529 (ND Ill 1997), not published.   Plaintiffs brought a declaratory judgment action seeking a determination of their obligations and duties to defendant, a doctor who was sued by his patient. The patient alleged several counts against the doctor, including that the doctor was negligent in failing to properly diagnose and treat her and that he induced her into "a meretricious, unethical and dependent relationship with him, [and] engaged in physical and sexual acts which he knew were medically and therapeutically harmful and improper." The plaintiff, on receiving notice of the suit, notified the doctor that pursuant to the "undue familiarity exclusion" in the insurance policy, any award of damages would be denied indemnification and any amount expended in defense of the claim would be limited to $100,000. The doctor disagreed with plaintiff regarding the applicability and interpretation of the "undue familiarity" exclusion. Plaintiff filed an action seeking a declaratory judgment elucidating the boundaries of their duties and obligations to the defendant under the policy. The court's analysis began with its resolution of whether the term *claim* in the policy was ambiguous. The court concluded that the term *claim* referred only to those counts that allege undue familiarity. Therefore, the court held that the plaintiff is bound by the terms of the policy to defend against those counts in the suit that made no mention of any conduct that comes within the ambit of "undue familiarity," and consequently to defend against the suit in its entirety.

Franklin v. Professional Risk Management Services, Inc., 987 F Supp 71 (D Mass 1997).   The court held that under Massachusetts law, "undue-familiarity" exclusion in a psychiatrist's professional liability insurance policy barred coverage for psychiatrist's liability to patient arising out of consensual sexual relationship with a patient. 987 F Supp at 75–77.

American Home Assurance Co. v. Stephens, 130 F3d 123 (5th Cir 1997). Rehearing granted, 140 F3d 617 (5th Cir 1998).   Granting a petition for rehearing, the 5th Circuit court withdrew its previously issued opinion that a malpractice policy provision that limits recovery for nonsexual malpractice claims where sexual misconduct is also alleged violates Texas public policy. The court concluded that certification of the question to the Texas Supreme Court was appropriate.

Chicago Insurance Co. v. Materola, 955 P2d 982 (Ariz CtApp Div 1 1998). Patient filed a claim against her psychologist alleging professional negligence, a number of intentional torts, and statutory claims. The patient also alleged a negligence claim against the psychologist's wife. The plaintiff agreed to defend the psychologist but reserved its right to deny coverage based on policy language and various exclusions. The patient won a judgment against the psychologist and his wife and agreed not to execute her judgment against them in exchange for an assignment of their rights against the various insurance companies. The plaintiff filed its declaratory action, seeking a determination that its policy did not cover the patient's claims against the psychologist and his wife. The court held that a sexual acts exclusion provision in the psychologist's professional liability policy barred coverage for professional negligence, intentional tort, and statutory claims arising from the psychologist's sexual relationship with the former patient. 955 P2d at 984–987.

St. Paul Fire and Marine v. Gold, 149 F3d 1191. 1998 WL 327892 (10th Cir [Okla]), **unpublished disposition.** A patient filed a civil action against her psychologist in Oklahoma state district court, alleging that the doctor carelessly and negligently failed to use the proper standard of care in his therapy and counseling of her. Plaintiff, the psychologist's insurance company, filed a declaratory judgment action requesting a declaration that it had no duty to defend or indemnify the defendant because of the "sexual activity or contact" exclusion provision in the insurance policy. The court held that the exclusion provision was not ambiguous and that the alleged acts of professional misconduct were inextricably linked with the sexual activity and that coverage was precluded.

Endnotes

1. Although some cases involve therapists and patients of the same sex, the vast majority of reported cases deal with a male physician's sexual abuse of his female patient. Accordingly, for the purposes of this chapter, we will illustrate our examples using this most common scenario and speak of the male psychiatrist and his female patient.

2. 22 Am Jur 2nd *Damages* § 733 (1988).

3. See *Govar v. Chicago Insurance Co.*, 879 F2d 1581 (8th Cir 1989) ($342,000 verdict for plaintiff). Jorgenson et al. point out several psychotherapist malpractice cases in which damage awards have exceeded a million dollars. L. Jorgenson, S. Bishing, and P. Sutherland, *Therapist-Patient Sexual Exploitation and Insurance Liability*, 28 Tort & Insurance Law Journal 595, 599 n. 26 (1992).

4. A very small number of physicians decide to "go bare" by refusing to purchase any liability insurance and transferring assets to family members. Such tactics "make it financially pointless for a patient to sue for malpractice." Kenneth S. Abraham and Paul C. Weiler, *Enterprise Medical Liability and the Evolution of the American Health Care System*, 108 Harvard Law Review 381, 403 n. 81 (1994).

5. The term "bedpan insurer" is somewhat derisive. The metaphor seems to be that of a convenient but limited accommodation instead of the fully equipped facility.

6. R. Z. Folman, *Therapist-Patient Sex: Attraction and Boundary Problems*, 28 Psychotherapy 168 (Spring 1991).

7. Ibid.

8. L. Jorgenson, S. Bishing, and P. Sutherland, *Therapist-Patient Sexual Exploitation and Insurance Liability*, 28 Tort & Insurance Law Journal 595, 601 (1992) (citing *St. Paul Fire and Marine Insurance Company v. Mitchell*, 296 SE2d 126, 129 [GaApp 1992]).

9. For example, *Niedzielski v. St. Paul Fire and Marine Insurance Co.*, 589 A2d 130 (NH 1991).

10. For example, *St. Paul Fire and Marine Insurance Co. v. Shernow*, 610 A2d 1281 (Conn 1992) (dentist's sexual abuse of sedated patient so intertwined with and inseparable from negligent administration of sedative that insurer must extend coverage); *Snyder v. Major*, 789 F Supp 646 (SDNY 1992) (no coverage for plastic surgeon who raped sedated patient). But see *Lindheimer v. St. Paul Fire and Marine Insurance Co.*, 634 So2d 636 (Fla App 3 Dist 1994) (dentist who sexually abused sedated patient not covered under generic policy providing for coverage of professional services provided or which should have been provided).

11. 436 SW2d 753 (Mo 1968) (generic policy covers psychiatrist who induced his patient, after she professed her love for him, to file for divorce, move into an apartment above his office, engage in sexual relations, and invest with him in a farm—to which she later moved and at which the psychiatrist made her work as part of her therapy).

12. See *Zipkin v. Freeman*, 436 SW2d 753 (Mo 1968); *Simmons v. United States*, 805 F2d 1363 (9th Cir 1986); *Love v. St. Paul Fire and Marine Insurance Co.*, 459

NW2d 698 (Minn 1990); *St. Paul Fire and Marine Insurance Co. v. D.H.L.*, 459 NW2d 704 (Minn 1990).

13. See, for example, *Washington Insurance Guarantee Association v. Hicks*, 744 P2d 625, 627–628 (Wash App 1987) (chiropractor's sexual intercourse with patient in office not covered by generic policy covering medical incident).

14. *Vigilant Insurance Co. v. Employers Insurance of Wausau*, 626 F Supp 262 (SDNY 1986).

15. Ibid. at 266.

16. Ibid.

17. Ibid. at 264.

18. Ibid. at 266.

19. *Love v. St. Paul Fire and Marine Insurance Co.*, 459 NW2d 698, 702 (Minn 1990).

20. See *Love v. St. Paul Fire and Marine Insurance Co.*, 459 NW2d 698, 701 (Minn 1990) ("As we have noted, the professional services provided by a therapist require him to enter into a therapeutic alliance with the patient that invariably induces love-transference. Transference, of course, occurs at times in other relationships including that of medical doctor and patient, but the therapist alone elicits transference as a regular, accepted part of his practice in treating marital and sexual disorders.").

21. However, if sexual contact occurred between a patient and a biologically oriented psychiatrist whose professional relationship with the patient extended no further than brief meetings to adjust antidepressant or antipsychotic medication, the court might find no transference. See *Love v. St. Paul Fire and Marine Insurance Co.*, 459 NW2d 698, 702 (Minn 1990) ("We suppose a therapist might take sexual advantage of a patient without transference being present. In such a case, much like the medical doctor in Smith, the sexual conduct might well lie outside professional services.").

22. *L.L. v. Medical Protective Co.*, 362 NW2d 174, 178 (Wis App 1984).

23. See *Frankenmuth Mutual Insurance Co. v. Kompus*, 354 NW2d 303, 308 (Mich App 1984) ("engaging in sexual acts with a patient supports a malpractice claim by the patient. . . . Over prescription of drugs may also support such a claim."); *L.L. v. Medical Protective Co.*, 362 NW2d 174, 178 (Wis App 1984) (psychiatrist's malpractice is a departure from the proper standard of medical practice—a departure no different from the "improper administration of a drug or a defective operation.").

24. *St. Paul Fire and Marine Insurance Company v. D.H.L.*, 459 NW2d 701.

25. *St. Paul Fire and Marine Insurance Company v. D.H.L.*, 459 NW2d 704, 706 (Minn 1990).

26. *St. Paul Fire and Marine Insurance Company v. D.H.L.*, 459 NW2d 698, 703 (Minn 1990) (Coyne, J., dissenting).

27. See, for example, *Simmons v. United States*, 805 F2d 1363 (9th Cir 1986); *Vigilant Insurance Co. v. Kambly*, 319 NW2d 382, 385 (Mich App 1982). See also *Love v. St. Paul Fire and Marine Insurance Co.*, 459 NW2d 698, 701 (Minn 1990) ("[T]he therapist must both encourage transference and discourage certain aspects of it. This may be difficult to do and present an occupational risk. The therapeutic alliance in this situation gives rise to a duty, imposed by professional standards of

care as well as by ethical standards of behavior, to refrain from a personal relationship with the patient, whether during or outside therapy sessions . . . .").
28. *St. Paul Fire and Marine Insurance Co. v. Vigilant Insurance Co.*, 919 F2d 235, 238
    (4th Cir 1990).
29. N. Gartrell, J. Herman, S. Olarte, M. Feldstein, and R. Localio, *Psychiatrist-Patient
    Sexual Contact: Results of a National Survey, I. Prevalence*, 143 Am J Psychiatry
    1126 (1986).
30. *Mazza v. Huffaker*, 300 SE2d 833 (NC App 1983).
31. Ibid. at 837–838.
32. Ibid. at 836.
33. Ibid. at 838 [emphasis added].
34. See, for example, *Vigilant Insurance Co. v. Kambly*, 319 NW2d 382, 384 (Mich App
    1982) (legal expenses incurred by psychiatrist accused of sexual misconduct cov-
    ered by malpractice policy despite exclusion for "legal expense incurred due to al-
    leged criminal act").
35. The Common Law 3 (1881).
36. See, for example, *Vigilant Insurance Co. v. Kambly*, 319 NW2d 382 (Mich App
    1982); *Vigilant Insurance Co. v. Employers Insurance of Wausau*, 626 F Supp 262
    (SDNY 1986).
37. *Vigilant Insurance Co. v. Employers Insurance of Wausau*,626 F Supp at 267 (SDNY
    1986).
38. *Vigilant Insurance Co. v. Kambly*, 319 NW2d 382, 385 (Mich App 1982).
39. Ibid. at 384.
40. Ibid. at 385.
41. Ibid.
42. *Roy v. Hartogs*, 381 NYS2d 587, 591 (App Div 1976) (Riccobono, J., dissenting).
43. See, for example, *Noto v. St. Vincent's Hospital and Medical Center of New York*, 537
    NYS2d 446, 448–449 (1988).
44. *Vigilant Insurance Co. v. Kambly*, 319 NW2d 384.
45. Ibid. at 384–385.
46. "Psychiatrists and Neurologists Professional Liability Policy," issued by the Amer-
    ican Home Assurance Company, Form #51481, p. 3 (June 1991).
47. "Description of Coverage," American Psychiatric Association–sponsored Profes-
    sional Liability Insurance Program, p. 5.
48. *LaPoint v. Richards*, 66 Wash 2d 585, 594–595, 403 P2d 889, 895 (1965) (citations
    omitted).
49. *Brown v. Snohomish County Physicians Corporation*, 845 P2d 334, 338 (Wash
    1993).
50. See Alan A. Stone, *Law, Psychiatry, and Morality* 191–192 (1984).
51. "Approximately 90% of the victims of sexual misconduct on the part of therapists
    are women." *American Home Assurance Company v. Cohen*, 881 P2d 1001, 1006
    (Wash 1994) (citing Jacqueline Bouhoutsos et al., *Sexual Intimacy Between Psycho-
    therapists and Patients*, 14 Professional Psychology: Research & Practice No. 2
    185, 188 [1983]; Kenneth S. Pope and Valerie A. Vetter, *Prior Therapist-Patient
    Sexual Involvement Among Patients Seen by Psychologists*, 28 Psychotherapy 429,
    433 [1991]).

52. "The theory of disparate impact is generally applied in the employment setting and differs from disparate treatment. In the latter case, an individual would be treated differently because of sex, race, age or some other improper differentiation. In cases involving disparate impact a facially neutral policy or practice would result in discrimination because of sex, race, age or other improper distinction." *American Home Assurance Co. v. Cohen*, 881 P2d 1001, 1006 (Wash 1994) (citation omitted).
53. *American Home Assurance Co. v. Cohen*, 881 P2d 1001 (Wash 1994).
54. Ibid. at 1003.
55. Ibid. at 1001.
56. Ibid. at 1007.
57. The *Cohen* court pointed out that some insurance coverage might be provided in the future, however: beginning in July 1995, Washington state law will require some health care providers to maintain a minimum level of malpractice insurance. Ibid at 1007, n. 19 (citing RCW 18.130.330 [Laws of 1994, ch. 102, s. 1, p. 559]). This new law might change future courts' analysis of the public policy of the state.
58. Ibid. at 1008.
59. Ibid.
60. *American Home Assurance Company v. Cohen*, 815 F Supp 365, 371 (WDWash 1993) (citing *American Home Assurance Company v. Oraker*, No. 90CV6483 [Colo DistCt March 5, 1992], Exh. C, Boyle's Dec., docket no. 12).
61. *American Home Assurance Co. v. Cohen*, 815 F Supp 365, 373 (WDWash 1993).
62. *American Home Assurance Co. v. Cohen*, 881 P2d 1001 (Wash 1994).
63. Ibid. at 1009.
64. Ibid.
65. Ibid.
66. Ibid.
67. Ibid. at 1010.
68. Ibid.
69. 1994 WL 543468, *9 (NDIll).
70. 740 Ill Comp Stat 140/1 et seq. (1989).
71. 1994 WL 543468, *9 (NDIll).
72. "Description of Coverage," American Psychiatric Association–sponsored Professional Liability Insurance Program, p. 5.
73. Insurance companies often go to court to resolve the question of which policy provides coverage. See, for example, *Frankenmuth Mutual Insurance Co. v. Kompus*, 354 NW2d 303 (Mich App 1984).
76. *Hartogs v. Employers Mutual Liability Insurance Co. of Wisconsin*, 391 NYS2d 962 (AppDiv 1977).
75. *Vigilant Insurance Co. v. Kambly*, 319 NW2d 382, 385 (Mich App 1982).
76. "Description of Coverage," American Psychiatric Association–sponsored Professional Liability Insurance Program.
77. It is my (AAS) experience, based on numerous consultations by victims over the years, that false claims of sexual misconduct are extremely rare. Accordingly, patients who have consulted me are usually considered to be reporting instances of

actual abuse. See Alan A. Stone, *Law, Psychiatry, and Morality* 192 (American Psychiatric Press, 1984).

78. There exists a complicated set of legal doctrines of corporate liability, respondeat superior, and other forms of vicarious liability that are related to the responsibilities of employers for their employees. Although it is beyond the scope of this chapter to explore such doctrines, it should be noted that one court has found as a matter of law that a psychotherapist who engages in sexual relations with a patient cannot be said to operate outside the scope of his employment, and therefore the therapist's employer may be liable for such actions. *St. Paul Fire and Marine Insurance Company v. Downs*, 617 NE2d 338 (Ill App 1 Dist 1993).

79. 42 USCA § 11111 et seq. (1990).
80. Ibid.
81. Ibid.
82. Ibid.
83. 607 NYS2d 296 (AD 1 Dept 1994).
84. Ibid. at 297.
85. Ibid.
86. Ibid.
87. Ibid. at 298.
88. Ibid. at 298–299.
89. See, for example, 28 Trial News & Trends (October 1992).
90. Personal clinical experience of AAS.
91. See *Riley v. Presnell*, 565 NE2d 780, 784 (Mass 1991).
92. Linda Jorgenson and Rebecca M. Randles, *TIME OUT: The Statute of Limitations and Fiduciary Theory in Psychotherapist Sexual Misconduct Cases*, unpublished paper, p. 37.
93. See ibid. at 39–69.
94. *Mansfield v. Watson*, 990 F2d 1258, 1993 WL 74374 (9th Cir[Wash]).
95. Ibid. at *2.
96. *Roe v. Jefferson*, 1994 WL 87763 (Tenn).
97. Ibid. at *6 (Tenn).
98. 453 Supp 765 (ED Pa 1978).
99. 805 F2d 1363, 1367 (9th Cir 1986).
100. Ibid. at 1367–1368.
101. *Riley v. Presnell*, 565 NE2d 780 (Mass 1991).
102. See, for example, L. Jorgenson, S. Bishing, and P. Sutherland, *Therapist-Patient Sexual Exploitation and Insurance Liability*, 28 Tort & Insurance Law Journal, 595, 608–614 (1992).
103. Data supplied by Alan Levenson, M.D., of the Psychiatrist's Purchasing Group.
104. Ibid.
105. Alan Levenson, personal communication, March 1995.
106. J. M Epstein, *The Exploitative Psychotherapist Defendant*, 25 Trial 53, 57 (1989) [emphasis added].
107. Ibid.
108. "Description of Coverage," American Psychiatric Association–sponsored Professional Liability Insurance Program, p. 5.

109. L. Jorgenson, S. Bishing, and P. Sutherland, *Therapist-Patient Sexual Exploitation and Insurance Liability*, 28 Tort & Insurance Law Journal 595, 608 (1992).

110. 645 F Supp 1440 (ND Cal 1986).

111. L. Jorgenson, S. Bishing, and P. Sutherland, *Therapist-Patient Sexual Exploitation and Insurance Liability*, 28 Tort & Insurance Law Journal 595, 608 (1992).

112. Ibid. at 610.

113. *Cranford Insurance Co. v. Allwest Insurance Co.*, 645 F Supp 1444 .

114. Ibid. (citing *State Farm Mutual Automobile Insurance Co. v. Partridge*, 514 P2d 123, 126 (Cal 1973).

115. 817 F Supp 861, 865 (D Hawaii 1993).

116. Ibid.

117. 879 F2d 1581 (8th Cir 1989).

118. Ibid at 1583.

119. Ibid at 1582.

120. 22 Am Jur 2d *Damages* § 23 (1988).

121. Ibid. at § 26.

122. Ibid. at § 733.

123. *Roy v. Hartogs*, 381 NYS2d 587, 589 (App Div 1976).

124. Ibid.

125. *Mazza v. Medical Mutual Life Insurance Co. of North Carolina*, 319 SE2d 217, 218 (NC 1984).

126. Ibid.

127. *Public Service Mutual Insurance Company v. Goldfarb*, 425 NE2d 810, 814 (NY 1981).

128. Ibid. at 814. As mentioned above, New York has distinguished between intentional conduct and intent to injure. Thus the *Goldfarb* court went on to state that a finding that the dentist intended to injure his patient would preclude insurance coverage of an award of both compensatory and punitive damages. To permit such an award would "violate 'the fundamental principle that no one shall be permitted to take advantage of his own wrong.' " Ibid.

129. L. Jorgenson, S. Bishing, and P. Sutherland, *Therapist-Patient Sexual Exploitation and Insurance Liability*, 28 Tort & Insurance Law Journal 595, 614 (1992).

130. *St. Paul Fire and Marine Insurance Company v. D.H.L.*, 459 NW2d at 701–702.

131. See *Chicago Insurance Co. v. Griffin*, 817 F Supp 861 (D Hawaii 1993); *Cranford Insurance Co. v. Allwest Insurance Co.*, 645 F Supp 1440 (NDCal 1986); *Rivera v. Nevada Medical Liability Insurance Co.*, 814 P2d 71, 74 (Nev 1991).

132. See, for example, *Hartogs v. Employers Mutual Liability Insurance Co. of Wisconsin*, 391 NYS2d 962, 964 (AppDiv 1977); *L.L. v. Medical Protective Co.*, 362 NW2d 174, 179 (Wis App 1984); *St. Paul Fire and Marine Insurance Co. v. Love*, 447 NW2d 5, 10 (Minn App 1989).

133. For example, *American Home Assurance Co. v. Cohen*, 881 P2d 1001, 1007–1009 (Wash 1994).

134. Ibid. at 1007 (citations omitted).

135. Ibid.

136. See *American Home Assurance Co. v. Cohen*, 881 P2d 1001, 1007 n. 19 (Wash 1994) (citing RCW 18.130.330 [Laws of 1994, ch. 102, s. 1, p. 559]).

137. For example, Cal Bus & Prof Code § 729(a), (c)(1)(West Supp 1991); 740 Ill Comp Stat 140/1 et seq. (1989).

138. See Michael T. Borruso, *Sexual Abuse by Psychotherapists: The Call for a Uniform Criminal Statute,* 17 Am J L & Med 289 (1991).

139. 60 ALR 5th 239 Vol 60 (1998) Westlaw Sect II (A).

140. L. Jorgenson, S. Bishing, and P. Sutherland, *Therapist-Patient Sexual Exploitation and Insurance Liability,* 28 Tort and Insurance Law Journal 595, 608 (1992).

SECTION II

Ethical and Regulatory Issues

4

SEXUAL MISCONDUCT, THE AMERICAN PSYCHIATRIC ASSOCIATION, AND THE AMERICAN MEDICAL ASSOCIATION

Ethics and Practice

Elissa P. Benedek, M.D., and David Wahl, M.D.

Case 1

Dr. Jane Smith, a child psychiatrist, met former patient Allen Jones in the supermarket. Allen was 16 years old when Dr. Smith treated him for depression after his parents died in an accident. Five years later, after this chance meeting, Allen called Dr. Smith to express his gratitude and invited her to observe a performance of his university theater group. He suggested that they meet after the performance for a drink. Dr. Smith agreed. She was pleased that her former patient had seemingly shaken off his grief and depression and was pursuing a career in acting. Subsequent to their encounter in the Green Room, Allen began to call Dr. Smith and asked her to go out with him. Dr. Smith was tempted and wondered what to do. Clearly, in her opinion, Allen was now a competent adult, able to make his own choices. A May-December relationship seemed flattering.

Case 2

Dr. James Young, a family physician, treated the Miller family for minor illnesses. He last treated Julie Miller when she was 18. Five years later, Julie and Dr. Young met at a football game.

Dr. Young found her attractive and wanted to ask her out. He was no longer her treating physician, and she was a consenting, competent adult with no history of psychiatric or psychological problems. Does the nature of the transference and the power disparity inherent in a psychiatric, therapeutic relationship apply to a family doctor?

Case 3

Dr. Rose Reed was Dr. Michael Green's training supervisor. Dr. Green, a child psychiatry fellow, asked Dr. Reed out to dinner. They were almost peers, but Dr. Reed hesitated. Dinner seemed innocuous, but what might it lead to? Is it ethical for a supervisor to engage in an intimate relationship with a consenting trainee? What about five years after training has ended?

Case 4

Dr. Merle George runs an anxiety disorders clinic and sees patients in brief consultation for other psychiatrists at the university. Dr. George evaluated Mr. Thomas Simpson in one brief session and referred him back to his treating psychiatrist with medication recommendations. Mr. Simpson, a successful businessman about Dr. George's age, called her to express his satisfaction with the consultation and suggested that they meet for dinner and drinks. As she considered the lack of suitable available men in her small community and Mr. Simpson's obvious attractions, she was tempted to say yes. Should a psychiatrist engage in an intimate relationship with a patient he or she has seen briefly for a psychopharmacological consultation?

Case 5

Dr. Peter Rembis is the psychiatrist of 23-year-old Gina Neville, a college graduate, who lives on her own. Dr. Rembis met Miss Neville's divorced mother at a community function and a week later asked her for a date. Since Miss Neville was an adult and her mother was not involved in her treatment in any way, he saw nothing wrong with his action. Is it ethical for a psychiatrist to date a patient's relative?

As these examples show, making ethical judgments about possible boundary violations can be quite complex. Such judgments often fall in a gray area for which formal codes of ethics can be useful reference tools for guiding professional conduct and making it possible to pass on professional standards of behavior to trainees.

Most physicians adhere to one or more sets of ethics codes, depending on the professional organizations to which they belong. For example, for psychiatrists these include the American Medical Association's "Principles of Medical Ethics" (American Medical Association 1996), the American Psychiatric Association's *Principles of Medical Ethics With Annotations Especially Applicable to Psychiatry* (American Psychiatric Association 1998), the American Academy of Child Psychiatry's *Principles of Practice for Child and Adolescent Psychiatry* (American Academy of Child Psychiatry 1998), and the American Academy of Psychiatry and the Law's *Ethical Guidelines for the Practice of Forensic Psychiatry* (American Academy of Psychiatry and the Law 1991).

Because the organizations that promulgate these ethics codes are voluntary membership organizations and, as such, cannot take disciplinary action against nonmembers, the codes are binding on members only. However, the codes may be used by courts and licensure boards in cases involving potential violations of prevailing medical ethics or practice standards.

In general, the codes are written as guidelines for professional conduct to be applied by individual practitioners in a wide variety of situations. In the case of sexual misconduct, however, the codes are explicit;
they leave no doubt that sexual activity between a physician and a patient is always unethical. The American Psychiatric Association's code
goes one step further by stating unequivocally that sexual activity between a psychiatrist and a former patient is always unethical. Many
states now have laws that back up these professional standards with
civil and/or criminal sanctions (see Bloom et al., Chapter 5; and Robinson, Chapter 6, in this volume).

History of Medical Ethics

Our modern ethical codes have their beginnings in ancient prayers and
incantations that sought inspiration, courage, and help in medical de-
terminations from the deities. The emphasis was on honor, trust, and
moral obligation. Most historians trace the formal roots of medical ethics to the Hippocratic Oath, a brief statement of principles, conceived in
Greece probably during the 5th century B.C. It protected the rights of
patients and appealed to the nobler instincts of physicians without imposing sanctions or penalties on them. While other civilizations developed their own principles, the Oath of Hippocrates has remained an
expression of ideal conduct for physicians and the basis for the contemporary practice of medicine in western cultures. In it are a series of
rules (not guidelines) that are similar in content, if not form, to current
standards (Moore 1978). Among these rules are preservation of patient
confidentiality, avoidance of sexual contact, and protection of patients
from harm. Allegedly, Greek physicians of Hippocrates' time ignored
the oath.

After Hippocrates, the most significant contribution to medical ethics in the West was made by Thomas Percival, an English physician/
philosopher and writer. In 1803, he published *Medical Ethics,* on
which the American Medical Association based its first officially
adopted code of ethics.

At the first official meeting of the American Medical Association
(AMA) in Philadelphia in 1847, two principal items of business were
the establishment of a code of ethics and the creation of requirements

for medical education. The AMA's ethics code (American Medical Association 1996) (see Appendix 4–1) underwent major revisions in 1903, 1912, and 1947. In 1955, an unsuccessful attempt was made to distinguish medical ethics from matters of etiquette. In 1977 the AMA's "Principles of Medical Ethics" were again revised in an attempt to clarify and update the language, to eliminate references to gender, and to seek a balance between professional standards and contemporary legal standards. In 1990 a companion code, "Fundamental Elements in the Patient-Physician Relationship," was produced by the AMA's Council on Ethical and Judicial Affairs and is now contained in the current edition of the *Code of Medical Ethics.*

In 1973, the American Psychiatric Association (APA) published its first edition of *Principles of Medical Ethics With Annotations Especially Applicable to Psychiatry* (American Psychiatric Association 1998) (see Appendix 4–2). The APA's code is primarily an elaboration of the AMA "Principles of Medical Ethics," based on the view that psychiatrists, as physicians, were bound by the AMA "Principles of Medical Ethics."

Over the years, the APA's Ethics Committee has received requests for opinions on the handling of ethics complaints and on the ethics of specific behavior, practices, and conduct of members and provides consultation to members by publishing its opinions. Such opinions have been published in 1979, 1983, 1985, 1989, 1992, 1993, and 1995. Unlike the principles, the opinions do not represent official APA positions. They provide an interpretation of the principles in the light of contemporary ethical problems.

In 1980, the Council of the American Academy of Child and Adolescent Psychiatry (AACAP) adopted its code of ethics (American Academy of Child Psychiatry 1998), recognizing that a code of ethics could not possibly address all issues; instead, it was seen as a dynamic document subject to growth, revision, and modification. The code emphasizes that the services of child and adolescent psychiatrists are more often sought by patients' parents or guardians than by the children or adolescents themselves. It also recognizes that schools, community mental health centers, and child protection agencies are more likely to use the services of child psychiatrists than are individual children. Thus the code attempts to deal with problems of dual or triple agency. This code also explicitly forbids sexual contact between patient and therapist.

The American Academy of Psychiatry and the Law's (AAPL's) guidelines were developed specifically for forensic psychiatrists (American Academy of Psychiatry and the Law 1991). These guidelines are silent or are vague on issues for which the committee drafting the guidelines could not reach a consensus, a situation that often arises when dealing with areas of ethical concern where there are several "right answers." The AAPL guidelines are not subject to enforcement, and complaints of possible infractions are referred to the APA when the AAPL member is also an APA member. Additionally, ethics complaints filed against AAPL members who belong to the AACAP and not the APA are referred to that organization, which in turn refers complaints to the appropriate state licensing boards.

Other professional organizations have also developed ethics principles. These include the American Psychological Association, the American College of Physicians, the National Organization of Social Workers, and the National Organization of Forensic Social Work. The principles of these organizations are not discussed in this chapter.

Sexual Misconduct

Ethics procedures of the American Medical Association.   The AMA has issued two specific opinions dealing with sexual misconduct in the practice of medicine. The first opinion deals with sexual harassment and exploitation between medical supervisors and trainees (American Medical Association 1996, opinion 3.08). The opinion first defines sexual harassment as sexual advances, requests for sexual favors, and other verbal or physical conduct of a sexual nature when "(1) such conduct interferes with an individual's work or academic performance or creates an intimidating, hostile, offensive work or academic environment; or (2) accepting or rejecting such conduct affects employment decisions or academic evaluations concerning the individual. *Sexual harassment is unethical*" [emphasis added].

The opinion then goes on to discuss the differential in power between medical supervisors and medical trainees. "Sexual relationships between a medical trainee and a supervisor, even when consensual, *are not acceptable, regardless of the degree of supervision in any given situation*" [emphasis added] (American Medical Association 1996). Thus, depending on the circumstances, inviting a trainee out for dinner and a drink may be considered harassment.

The second opinion dealing with sexual misconduct is document 8.14, "Sexual Misconduct in the Practice of Medicine." This opinion states that "sexual contact that occurs concurrent with the physician-patient relationship constitutes sexual misconduct. Sexual or romantic interactions between physicians and patients detract from the goals of the physician/patient relationship and may exploit the vulnerability of the patient, may obscure the physician's objective judgment concerning the patient's health care, and ultimately may be detrimental to the patient's well-being."

The opinion also states that if a physician has any reason to believe that nonsexual contact with a patient may be perceived as or lead to sexual contact, the physician should avoid the nonsexual contact. The opinion adds, "At a minimum, a physician's ethical duty includes terminating the physician-patient relationship before initiating a dating, romantic, or sexual relationship with a patient." Thus, the family practitioner who repeatedly asks a patient for a date and begins to indicate a romantic interest may also be crossing an ethical boundary.

Finally, the opinion states, sexual or romantic relationships with *former patients* are unethical "if the physician uses or exploits trust, knowledge, emotions, or influence derived from the previous professional relationship" (American Medical Association 1996).

The judicial authority of the AMA is the Council on Ethical and Judicial Affairs, and its decisions are final. One of the Council's functions is to interpret the principles of medical ethics. Another function is to investigate general ethical conditions and make recommendations to the House of Delegates. The Council also receives appeals and complaints filed by physicians or associations who allege they have, because of color, creed, race, religion, ethnic origin, nationality, or gender, been unfairly denied membership in a component association. It determines the facts of the case and reports its findings to the House of Delegates. If the Council determines that the allegations are true, it "shall admonish, censure, or recommend to the House of Delegates that the constituent association involved be declared to no longer be a constituent member of the AMA."

The Council also can request that the AMA president appoint an investigative jury to handle complaints of unethical conduct that in its judgment are of greater than local concern. Investigative juries may submit formal charges to the president, who may then appoint a prosecutor to try the case before the Council on Ethical and Judicial Affairs on behalf of the AMA.

There is also an appeal and a disciplinary process. Section 120 of the AMA's bylaws provides that a member "may retain membership only as long as the provisions of the Constitution and Bylaws and Principles of Medical Ethics of the American Medical Association are complied with." Section 1.621 of the bylaws provides that the Council on Ethical and Judicial Affairs, after due notice and hearings, may *censure, suspend, or expel* any active, direct associate, affiliate, or honorary member of the AMA for an infraction of the constitution or bylaws or for a violation of the "Principles of Medical Ethics" of the AMA. Section 1.611 provides that the Council on Ethical and Judicial Affairs, after due notice and hearing, may *censure, suspend, or expel* an active constituent association for an infraction of the constitution or bylaws or for violation of the "Principles of Medical Ethics." The *Code of Medical Ethics* describes a series of steps, including rules for a statement of charges, notification, response, and hearings when there is an ethical charge against a member (American Medical Association 1996). Rule 13 concludes by saying, "The Council on Ethical and Judicial Affairs shall not be bound by technical, legal rules of evidence and takes up any evidence or information deemed relevant." A member may have legal counsel, and a member's legal counsel may cross-examine any witnesses who appear.

Ethics procedures of the American Psychiatric Association.   The Ethics Committee of the APA developed the procedures for handling complaints of unethical conduct. The procedures are *general guidelines recommended by the APA.* There are variations in the interpretation and execution of the approved procedures among the district branches. *There is no statute of limitations on unethical conduct.*

The APA has also published a pamphlet for patients who wish to complain to local district branch ethics committees, outlining the various steps in the procedure as they are detailed in the *Principles of Medical Ethics* (American Psychiatric Association 1998).

All formal complaints charging an APA member with unethical behavior must be made in writing, signed by the complainant, and addressed to the accused member's district branch or to the APA. It is important to emphasize that filing an ethics complaint with the APA does not have any immediate or direct effect on a physician's license to practice medicine. Unless state laws dictate otherwise, APA procedures provide for forwarding complaints to licensing boards only after a final decision is reached and then only if there is a sanction of suspension or expulsion. Other sanctions, such as admonishment (an informal warning or reprimand, a form of censure), are not necessarily reported to licensing boards. These sanctions may also be reported to the federal government via the National Practitioner Data Bank.

After receiving a written complaint, the district branch determines whether there are compelling reasons that it would not be the appropriate body to consider the complaint. If it believes it is not the appropriate body, the district branch writes to the chair of the APA Ethics Committee, requesting that it be excused and detailing the reasons for its request. The chair of the Ethics Committee then determines whether the district branch should be excused. If it is not excused, the district branch proceeds with the complaint. If it is excused, the chair appoints three APA fellows to serve as an ad hoc committee to conduct an investigation and render a decision. The appointment of an ad hoc committee to investigate a complaint is discouraged by the APA Ethics Committee, as it has been the experience of the APA that local decision making best serves the profession and patients.

Generally, after a district branch receives a written complaint of unethical conduct, the chair or another member of the district branch ethics committee contacts the complainant to discuss the complaint, evaluate all available information, and decide whether the complaint is true and, as stated, constitutes an ethics violation.

If the local ethics committee determines that a complaint does not involve questions of unethical behavior, the case is closed and the district branch so notifies the complainant. The complainant may still request a review of the district branch decision by writing to the APA secretary.

If the committee decides that an ethical violation *may* have occurred, however, both the complainant and accused member are notified in writing that an investigation has been opened. The accused member receives a copy of the complainant's letter and may respond to the allegations, either in writing or in person, to a member of the district branch's ethics committee. In addition, the ethics committee may ask to review any relevant evidence, such as records of psychiatric treatment and bills.

The ethics committee then decides whether a formal hearing is warranted. If the possibility exists that the member might be sanctioned on the basis of a complaint, he or she will be given the option of a formal hearing in which all the charges and evidence of the case will be presented to the ethics committee or to a small subgroup of that committee. The complainant has a right to be present at the hearing and to testify against the psychiatrist. The psychiatrist has an opportunity to present a defense.

The district branch then conducts what is intended to be a comprehensive and fair hearing unless the accused psychiatrist has voluntarily waived his or her right to a hearing, or the district branch has determined that there is no violation. At least 30 days beforehand, the accused member is notified of the hearing by certified mail, as is the complainant. Attendance at these hearings varies somewhat among APA's district branches. Those present might include the accused member; the complainant; members of the ethics committee; an attorney representing the accused psychiatrist; a complainant's advocate, friend, and/or attorney; an attorney representing the district branch; witnesses on behalf of either the complainant or the accused member; and administrative staff of the district branch. Most district branches attempt to comply with scheduling requests.

At the hearing, which is audiotaped, the complainant is asked to present his or her complaint to members of the ethics committee. Following the presentation, the accused physician or the accused member's attorney may cross-examine the complainant with the careful scrutiny of the hearing office to ensure that such cross-examination is done with dignity and respect for the complainant and stays focused on the relevant material. If the chair determines that such cross-examination would be harmful to the complainant, written questions or elimination of such cross-examination is possible. Following the complainant's testimony and cross-examination, the complainant may be allowed to hear the accused member's testimony, but this practice varies among district branches.

The ethics committee then makes a recommendation in writing, including a statement of the basis for the recommendation. This recommendation is referred to the district branch, which decides whether an ethics violation has occurred, and, if so, what sanction is appropriate. The district branch then decides on one of four possible sanctions:

1) admonishment—an informal warning; 2) reprimand—a formal sanction; 3) suspension—for a period not to exceed 5 years; or 4) expulsion. In addition to these, a district branch may impose certain conditions, such as educational or supervisory requirements on a suspended member.

The district branch's council then forwards the recommendations to the APA's Ethics Committee for review. Following that review, the district branch makes a final decision and notifies the accused member. The member has a right to appeal that decision before the APA Ethics Appeals Board. The appeal is generally based on one or more of the following criteria: 1) that there have been significant procedural irregularities or deficiencies in the case; 2) that the Principles of Medical Ethics have been improperly applied; 3) that the findings or sanction imposed by the district branch is not supported by substantial evidence; or 4) that substantial new evidence has called into question the findings and conclusions of the district branch.

Various procedures apply with regard to the hearing and the Ethics Appeals Board that will not be detailed here. However, after hearing the appeal and reviewing the record, the Ethics Appeals Board may take any one of the following actions: 1) affirm the decision, including the sanction imposed by the district branch; 2) affirm the decision but alter the sanction imposed by the district branch; 3) reverse the decision of the district branch and terminate the case; or 4) remand the case to the district branch with specific instructions regarding what further information or action is necessary.

Finally, if the decision is to expel a member, the APA's Board of Trustees must review the decision and can affirm it, impose a lesser sanction, or remand the case back to the Ethics Appeals Board. In addition to a letter to the accused member, the district branch sends a letter to the complainant detailing the final findings of the complaint and sanctions as appropriate. District branches are encouraged to prepare such letters with sensitivity to the often long delay the complainant must endure awaiting a final decision.

To ensure proper protection of the public, there are times when disclosure of the identity of the accused member may be essential; as such, the name of any member who is expelled from the APA for an ethics violation, along with an explanation of the nature of the violation, is reported in the APA's newspaper, *Psychiatric News*, the district branch newsletter or any other usual means of communication with APA membership, and local newspapers. In addition, the information is reported to the medical licensing authority in all states in which the member is licensed. It is also reported to any foreign psychiatric society or association to which the member belongs. Likewise, the name of any member who is suspended from the APA, along with an explanation of the nature of the violation, may be reported in *Psychiatric News* and to the medical licensing authority.

The names of expelled and suspended members are also reported to the National Practitioner Data Bank, which went into effect September 1, 1990. The data bank contains records of medical professionals and dentists who have been successfully sued (even if settled), whose licenses have been revoked or suspended, or who have been sanctioned by a hospital medical group or health plan with a peer review system.

The name of any member who resigns from the APA after an ethics complaint is filed against him or her is also reported in *Psychiatric News* and in the member's district branch newsletter. The name of a member against whom an ethics complaint is filed within 90 days after the member submits a resignation may be reported to the membership and to the National Practitioner Data Bank. The APA Board of Trustees or, after approval by the APA Ethics Committee, a district branch's governing council may report an ethics charge or a decision finding that a member has engaged in unethical conduct to any medical licensing authority, medical society, hospital clinic, or other institutions or persons where such disclosure is deemed appropriate to protect the public.

Despite the clear prohibitions against sexual activity with patients and former patients, sexual misconduct continues to be one of the leading causes of ethics complaints filed against APA members. Of the 113 APA members who were suspended or expelled from the organization in the last decade, most were found to have committed sexual transgressions. This figure undoubtedly represents only the tip of the iceberg, because many cases of sexual misconduct still go unreported.

Sexual Activity Between a Patient and Psychiatrist

Sexual activity between a patient and a psychiatrist is always unethical. Psychiatrists accused of such behavior have attempted to defend themselves in a variety of ways, including attacking the victim as a liar or seducer, asserting that the victim was psychologically impaired previously or that the psychological impairment was not a result of the sexual activity, or claiming that the affair between the psychiatrist and the patient was "true love."

Such defenses rarely, if ever, are viable. As the public, APA members, and members of the local and national ethics committees have become increasingly educated and sophisticated, these defenses have been less frequently advanced, and when they are advanced, they are less frequently accepted.

More recently, controversy has centered around sexual activity with former patients. The APA's earlier ethics guideline, which stated that sexual activity with a former patient "almost always is unethical," was seen as ambiguous and as providing a loophole for psychiatrists to engage in an intimate relationship with a patient. In the late 1980s and early 1990s, the APA considered dropping "almost always" from the principle and unequivocally stating that sexual activity with former patients is unethical. The debate was long and acrimonious. Some insisted that "once a patient, always a patient," while others felt that there were gray areas, such as the psychopharmacologist who sees a patient for a one-time consultation. Some members feared that if some cases of sexual involvement with a patient were not considered unethical, it would suggest that the APA was inconsistent. Others felt that the change would represent a paternalistic denial of former patients' capacity to act as adults in deciding whether or not to enter into an intimate relationship.

Appelbaum and Jorgenson (1991) focused the debate when they proposed a 1-year waiting period between the termination of therapy and the initiation of sexual contact between patient and therapist. Admitting that such a proposal had its problems, the authors nevertheless argued that an absolute 1-year rule was reasonable. They adamantly stated that the goal of their proposal was not to "encourage sexual contact between psychotherapists and former patients"; but since intimate contact does occur, they felt the need for a workable policy to ensure that patients are not exploited and enforcement is consistent and fair.

Stimulated by reaction to Appelbaum and Jorgenson's article and by high-profile cases, the APA's Assembly of District Branches recommended a change in the ethics principle to declare sexual relations with former patients unethical. In July 1993, by a vote of 9–7, the Board of Trustees agreed. Continued debate around this change focuses on the changing role of psychiatrists in treatment relationships (e.g., psychopharmacological treatment, in which some argue that the transferential nature of the relationship is minimal).

Sexual exploitation of patients by psychiatrists became front-page news and the subject of a number of best-sellers during the past decade. As popular perceptions of physicians as flawless healers and women as powerless, hysterical fantasizers have changed, victims have become more willing to come forward to tell their stories and take action against the perpetrators.

In the aftermath of some of the more notorious of these cases and research indicating the pervasiveness of patient-therapist boundary violations, the APA clarified its ethics principles and made sanctions more stringent. Moreover, the APA, as well as the field of psychiatry, has taken steps to make ethics—especially pertaining to boundary violations—an integral part of psychiatry residency training and a major topic at the annual meeting.

Discussion

The cases presented at the beginning of this chapter illustrate some of the problematic situations regarding boundary violations that ethics committees have increasingly had to consider. All of the scenarios described are unethical.

The ethics principle in cases 1 and 4 is that for psychiatrists sexual activity with a former patient is always unethical, regardless of the length of time that has elapsed since treatment has ended. When asked whether there might be exceptions to this principle, the APA's Ethics Committee replied, "If a complaint that raises this issue is filed against a member psychiatrist, it becomes the responsibility of the district branch ethics committee to deal with that complaint by careful consideration of all the relevant facts, especially any evidence indicating exploitation of the former patient. The ethics committee will then determine whether the accused psychiatrist has behaved unethically."

Case 2 appears to be more complex because the physician interested in pursuing a relationship with a former patient is a family doctor, not a psychiatrist. Although there is no question that a psychiatrist in this situation would be acting unethically if he or she entered into an intimate relationship with a former patient, the AMA Code of Ethics states that such a relationship is unethical "if the physician uses or exploits trust, knowledge, emotions, or influence derived from the previous professional relationship." Thus, if the relationship were to sour, the former patient/girlfriend could have some basis to file ethics charges against the physician.

The psychiatrist in case 3 would be acting unethically if she accepted her trainee's invitation to dinner. They are not professional equals; she clearly holds the power in their current relationship and is in a position to affect his future. If she did become involved with her trainee, not only could she be brought up on ethics charges, but she also runs the risk of sexual harassment charges under federal law.

The psychiatrist in case 5 would be acting unethically by dating his patient's mother. Again, there is a power discrepancy in the relationship.

In psychiatry the current absolute prohibition against sexual activity between therapist and former patient is warranted. The risk of harm to individual therapists, patients, and the profession clearly outweighs any benefit. Furthermore, the fiduciary relationship between a profession and society and the parallel relationship between a therapist and a patient are jeopardized by such activity.

In tightening its ethics code with regard to sexual misconduct, the APA's deliberation was motivated by a triple interest to balance the special needs of patients, the public, and members. This is exemplified by the discussion to permit the publication of names of expelled members in *Psychiatric News* and their local newspapers. Some trustees and members of the APA's Ethics Committee believed that suspension and expulsion from a professional organization were sufficient punishment for offending members and that they ought not be shamed further by the publication of their names in newspapers or professional newsletters. They worried that suspension or expulsion might lead to self-harm. An equally vocal majority noted that it was important for the public to be protected and that publication would inform peers outside the small circle of the Ethics Committee about names and practices of offending psychiatrists. They agreed, however, that the salacious details of a psychiatrist's offending behavior would not be publicized.

In the coming decade, the entire ethics process itself—rather than just specific principles—may come under fire. As the costs for the fair and thorough investigation of ethics cases increase, along with concerns over an organization's potential liability for damaging the course of a member's career against whom the most severe sanctions are taken, some organizational leaders may believe it a sound fiduciary decision to leave the sanctioning of medical doctors to their respective licensing authorities (see Bloom et al., Chapter 5, in this volume).

Adding weight to this argument is the fact that the public does not appear to understand that membership in a professional organization is voluntary and can therefore be terminated at any time. If a person accused of unethical conduct never joins his or her professional organization or terminates membership during an investigation, the organization cannot take any action against that person. Complainants sometimes perceive this fact to indicate the organization's unwillingness to "police its own." Moreover, if ethics complaints were handled by the licensing authority only, complainants would not have to expend their resources on two—and sometimes more—fronts to achieve what they believe is justice. In the end, the loss or restriction of the license to practice one's livelihood rather than colleagues' censure has the longer-lasting impact.

On the other hand, it is my opinion that a professional organization that does not actively promote and enforce a code of ethical behavior is in danger of rapidly becoming a trade or guild organization, whose sole focus may be the economic well-being of its membership. Public opinion and professional responsibility and integrity dictate that a profession devote both its economic capital and membership resources to this difficult activity, which is crucial and necessary to professional survival and patient protection.

References

American Academy of Child Psychiatry: Principles of Practice for Child and Adolescent Psychiatry. Washington, DC, American Academy of Child Psychiatry, 1998
American Academy of Psychiatry and the Law: Ethical Guidelines for the Practice of Forensic Psychiatry. Washington, DC, American Academy of Psychiatry and the Law, 1991

American Association for Marriage and Family Therapy: AAMFT Code of Ethical Principles for Marriage and Family Therapists. Washington, DC, American Association for Marriage and Family Therapy, 1988

American Medical Association, Council on Ethical and Judicial Affairs: Code of Medical Ethics: Current Opinions With Annotations. Chicago, IL, American Medical Association, 1996

American Psychiatric Association: Principles of Medical Ethics With Annotations Especially Applicable to Psychiatry. Washington, DC, American Psychiatric Association, 1998

Appelbaum PS, Jorgenson LL: Psychotherapist-patient sexual contact after termination of treatment: an analysis and a proposal. Am J Psychiatry 148:1466–1473, 1991

Moore RA: Ethics in the practice of psychiatry—origins, functions, models, and enforcement. Am J Psychiatry 135:157–163, 1978

Appendix 4-1. The American Medical Association's Principles of Medical Ethics[1]

Preamble

The medical profession has long subscribed to a body of ethical statements developed primarily for the benefit of patients. As a member of this profession, a physician must recognize responsibility not only to patients, but also to society, to other health professionals, and to self. The following principles adopted by the American Medical Association are standards of conduct that define the essentials of honorable behavior for the physician.

    I. A physician shall be dedicated to providing competent medical service with compassion and respect for human dignity.

    II. A physician shall deal honestly with patients and colleagues and strive to expose those physicians deficient in character or competence, or who engage in fraud or deception.

    III. A physician shall respect the law and also recognize a responsibility to seek changes in those requirements which are contrary to the best interests of the patient.

    IV. A physician shall respect the rights of patients, of colleagues, and of other health professionals, and shall safeguard patient confidences within the constraints of the law.

    V. A physician shall continue to study, apply, and advance scientific knowledge, make relevant information available to patients, colleagues, and the public, obtain consultation, and use the talents of other health professionals when indicated.

    VI. A physician shall, in the provision of appropriate patient care, except in emergencies, be free to choose whom to serve, with whom to associate, and the environment in which to provide medical services.

    VII. A physician shall recognize a responsibility to participate in activities contributing to an improved community.

---

[1]Reprinted from American Medical Association: Code of Medical Ethics. Chicago, IL, American Medical Association, 1996. Used with permission.

Fundamental Elements of the Patient-Physician Relationship

Accompanying the AMA's principles of medical ethics are the fundamental elements of the patient-physician relationship.

1. The patient has the right to receive information from physicians and to discuss the benefits, risks, and costs of appropriate treatment alternatives. Patients should receive guidance from their physicians as to the optimal course of action. Patients are also entitled to obtain copies or summaries of their medical records, to have their questions answered, to be advised of potential conflicts of interest that their physicians might have, and to receive independent professional opinion.

2. The patient has the right to make decisions regarding the health care recommended by his or her physician. Accordingly, the patient may accept or refuse any recommended medical treatment.

3. The patient has the right to courtesy, respect, dignity, responsiveness, and timely attention to his or her needs.

4. The patient has the right to confidentiality. The physician should not reveal confidential communications or information without the consent of the patient, unless provided for by law or by the need to protect the welfare of the individual or the public interest.

5. The patient has the right to continuity of health care. The physician has an obligation to cooperate in the coordination of medically indicated care with other health care providers treating the patient. The physician may not discontinue treatment of a patient as long as further treatment is medically indicated without giving the patient sufficient opportunity to make alternative arrangements for care.

6. The patient has a basic right to have available adequate health care. Physicians, along with the rest of society, should continue to work toward this goal. Fulfillment of this right is dependent on society's providing resources so that no patient is deprived of necessary care because of an inability to pay for the care. Physicians should continue their traditional assumption of a part of the responsibility for the medical care of those who cannot afford essential health care.

Appendix 4–2. Excerpts From the American Psychiatric Association's Principles of Medical Ethics With Annotations Especially Applicable to Psychiatry[2]

In 1973, the APA first published the *Principles of Medical Ethics With Annotations Especially Applicable to Psychiatry.* Several revisions have followed, the most recent of which is the 1998 Edition. Although all of the principles may deal in some way with sexual exploitation, the following principles are the most relevant:

> **Section 1.**   *A physician shall be dedicated to providing medical service with compassion and respect for human dignity.*

Annotation 1.   The patient may place his/her trust in his/her psychiatrist knowing that the psychiatrist's ethics and professional responsibilities preclude his/her gratifying his/her own needs by exploiting the patient. The psychiatrist shall be ever vigilant about the impact that his/her conduct has upon the boundaries of the doctor/patient relationship and thus upon the well-being of the patient. These requirements become particularly important because of the essentially private, highly personal, and sometimes intensely emotional nature of the relationship established with the psychiatrist.[3]

> **Section 2.**   *A physician shall deal honestly with patients and colleagues and strive to expose those physicians deficient in character or confidence, or who engage in fraud or deception.*

Annotation 1.   The requirement that the physician conduct himself/herself with propriety in his/her profession and in all the actions of his/her life is especially important in the case of the psychiatrist because the patient tends to model his/her behavior after that of

---

[2]Reprinted with permission from the American Psychiatric Association. Copyright 1998 American Psychiatric Association.

[3]Thus, the psychiatrist who exploits a patient by borrowing money from the patient or entering into a business arrangement with a patient, or who sexually harasses or abuses a patient, is acting unethically.

his/her psychiatrist by identification. Further, the necessary intensity of the treatment relationship may tend to activate sexual and
other needs and fantasies on the part of both patient and psychiatrist,
while weakening the objectivity necessary for control. Additionally,
the inherent inequality in the doctor/patient relationship can lead to
exploitation of the patient. *Sexual activity with a current or former patient is unethical.*[4]

Annotation 2.   The psychiatrist should diligently guard against exploiting information furnished by the patient and should not use the
unique power afforded him/her by the psychotherapeutic situation
to influence the patient in any way not directly relevant to the treatment goals.

Annotation 5.   Psychiatric services, like all medical services, are dis-
pensed in the context of a contractual arrangement between the patient and the treating physician. The provisions of the contractual
arrangement which are binding on the physician as well as on the patient should be explicitly established.

Section 4.   *A physician shall respect the rights of patients, of colleagues, and of other health professionals and shall safeguard patient
confidences within the constraints of the law.*

Annotation 14.   Sexual involvement between a faculty member or supervisor and a trainee or student, in those situations in which an
abuse of power can occur, often takes advantage of inequalities in
the working relationship and may be unethical because (a) any treatment of a patient being supervised may be deleteriously affected; (b)
it may damage a trusting relationship between teacher and student;
and (c) teachers are important professional role models for their
trainees and affect their trainees' future professional behavior.

---

[4]Note that sexual activity with a *former* patient always is unethical. This portion of the
annotation has been hotly debated. Some APA members want the previous wording
"almost always" to be retained.

5

SEXUAL MISCONDUCT AND BOARDS OF MEDICAL EXAMINERS

Joseph D. Bloom, M.D., Mary H. Williams, M.S., J.D., John J. Ulwelling, M.A., and Harvey Klevit, M.D.

Was a 29-year-old Portland woman driven to suicide by her psychiatrist? The question may be impossible to answer. She left no note when she shot herself with a .38-caliber pistol and was found dead on June 26. But her sister and friends say that she was driven over the edge by a shrink whose license had just been suspended (because of sexual misconduct) by the state Board of Medical Examiners.

Willamette Week 1994

Recognizing that to practice medicine is not a natural right of any person but is a privilege granted by legislative authority, it is necessary in the interests of the health, safety, and welfare of the people of this state to provide for the regulation of its use, to the end that the public is protected from the practice of medicine by unauthorized or unqualified persons and from unprofessional conduct by persons licensed to practice under this chapter.

Oregon Revised Statutes, Chapter 677.015, 1993

We thank Ms. Chris Land for her help with data management on this chapter.

The practice of medicine is not a right; it is a privilege. Medical schools award professional degrees, but by granting a license to a physician medical boards translate that degree into a professional practice career. Other powerful deliberative bodies do not have the specific authority to terminate a physician's ability to practice his or her profession. For example, a court in a malpractice action may separate a physician from assets, or in a criminal conviction may restrict the physician's personal liberty. An ethics committee of a professional society may harm a physician's reputation with a recommendation that the physician be expelled from that society. However, only the medical board can terminate a physician's ability to practice medicine within the board's jurisdiction.

In this chapter we explore the role of medical boards in relation to the problem of sexual misconduct by physicians. We present data from several sources: two reviews of sexual misconduct complaints reported to the Oregon Board of Medical Examiners, and a national survey of medical boards focused on sexual misconduct. Discussion of these data will lead to an initial view of how these boards are discharging their responsibilities in relation to complaints of sexual misconduct.

The Oregon Board of Medical Examiners—Powers and Procedures

Although medical boards are not necessarily identical in their organization, the procedures of the Oregon board generally mirror those of medical boards across the country.

The Oregon Board of Medical Examiners is responsible for the licensing and discipline of certain health professionals, including physicians who by applying for an Oregon medical license have chosen to place themselves under the board's jurisdiction and to abide by its rules. The board's activities are governed by the Medical Practice Act, a section of Oregon statutes that regulates the practice of medicine, podiatry, and related medical services (Oregon 1993). A key section of this statute lists 27 grounds for suspending, revoking, or refusing to grant a medical license (Oregon 1993, § 190).

The board is composed of nine physicians and two lay members, appointed by the governor. Two major committees assist the board: the

Administrative Affairs Committee is responsible for review of applications for licensure, and the Investigative Committee reviews complaints made against licensed practitioners, medical and osteopathic physicians, podiatrists, physician assistants, acupuncturists, and advanced emergency technicians. Complaints are initially screened and investigated by staff members of the board. They refer possible statutory violations to the Investigative Committee, which determines whether the physician will be asked to appear for an interview to review the specific case(s) in question. At that meeting the physician may choose to be accompanied by legal counsel.

Following the interview, the Investigative Committee decides on a course of action. It may close the case, with or without a letter of concern to the physician, and/or recommend certain educational programs designed to improve the physician's quality of care. Participation in such programs does not constitute a disciplinary action and is not reportable to the public.

However, if there is a potential serious violation of the Medical Practice Act, the case is referred to the full board for further deliberation. The board may choose to close the case, or it may take an action against the physician's license, including suspension, fine, probation, or revocation. Physicians have a right to a formal administrative hearing. Based on the findings of the hearings officer, the board decides on disciplinary action, which may be appealed by the physician to the Oregon Court of Appeals.

Sexual Misconduct Complaints and the Oregon Board of Medical Examiners

Oregon statutes do not make specific mention of sexual misconduct by health professionals. The board has handled most sexual misconduct cases under the category of unprofessional or dishonorable conduct (Oregon 1993, § 190), although gross negligence, repeated acts of negligence, and habitual use of intoxicants have had relevance in some of these cases. Furthermore, unlike some jurisdictions, Oregon statutes do not specifically mandate reporting of sexual misconduct. However, there is a statutory provision mandating that licensed physicians must report other physicians to the board when there is a question that he or she "may be medically incompetent or is or may be guilty of unprofessional or dishonorable conduct or is or may be an impaired physician unable safely to engage in the practice of medicine" (Oregon 1993, § 415 [2]).

To examine the experience of the Oregon board in relation to complaints of sexual misconduct, we reviewed a recent article by Enbom and Thomas (1997) on sexual misconduct complaints between 1991 and 1995. We supplemented these findings with a previously unreported informal survey of similar complaints during an overlapping 3-year period, 1991–1993.

Enbom and Thomas (1997) reported that there were 100 complaints of alleged sexual misconduct filed against 80 licensees during their study period. The percentage of sexually related complaints ranged from 5.3% of total complaints in 1991, to 8.3% in 1994, to 4.3% in 1995. Most complaints (74%) were brought by patients and/or family members.

Each complaint was categorized according to three groups previously developed by the Medical Council of New Zealand: sexual impropriety, such as inappropriate comments (39% of complaints); sexual transgression, such as inappropriate touching (31% of complaints); and sexual violation, a sexual relationship with a patient (30% of complaints).

Enbom and Thomas found higher proportions of complaints filed against physicians who practiced family medicine, obstetrics/gynecology, and psychiatry. Both of the latter groups had significantly higher proportions of cases reported to the National Practitioner Data Bank after formal action had been taken by the Oregon board.

Because our informal study overlapped with the period studied by Enbom and Thomas (1997), we will use our data to amplify some of their findings.

Seventy-two licensees had sexually related complaints, including 60 M.D.s (83%), 9 D.O.s (12%), 1 acupuncturist, 1 podiatrist, and 1 physician's assistant. With the 3 nonphysicians dropped from the analysis, 67 (97%) of the physicians in the sample were male. They ranged in age from 33 to 83, with a mean age of 53. They had been in practice from 5 to 57 years, with an average of 25 years of practice. Ninety-three percent of the physicians in the sample were graduates of American medical schools, and 58% were board certified. This compares with approximately 71% of Oregon physicians who are board certified (H. Klevit, personal communication, 1994).

Most complaints (64%) were initiated by patients or relatives of patients; only 13% came from other providers. It is interesting to note, however, that the Oregon board routinely reviews all malpractice case claims and settlements, and four complaints (6%) came from a review of malpractice cases. During this period the board received no complaints from an ethics committee of any medical professional society. It is also important to note that 54% of the sample had prior board complaints, of which 41% were of a sexual nature.

Our data also emphasize that the board handles the different complaint categories in significantly different ways. Complaints involving inappropriate examination were terminated in more than 90% of cases at the Investigative Committee level, whereas cases involving sexual relations with patients were most often handled at the level of the full board. Forty-two percent of physicians charged with sexual relations with patients continued to practice, whereas 32% were no longer practicing. It is important to note that we categorized six cases in our review as representing possible paraphilia and that 50% of these cases reached the board level.

Table 5–1 summarizes the dispositions of sexual relations complaints by medical specialty. Because of the small numbers, we combined family practice, general practice, and internal medicine and labeled the category primary care. If we compare the primary care physicians with psychiatrists, a different pattern begins to emerge. Four (50%) of the eight psychiatrists were out of practice compared with one (14%) of the primary care group.

Table 5–1.   Dispositions of sexual relations complaints by specialty

| Specialty | Number (%) of dispositions | | |
| | Committee | Board | |
		Practice	No practice
Primary care	3 (43)	3 (43)	1 (14)
Psychiatry	2 (25)	2 (25)	4 (50)
Other	0	3 (75)	1 (25)

Sexual Misconduct and Boards of Medical Examiners— A National Survey

In January 1994 we surveyed all medical boards in the United States ($N = 65$). The survey was designed to provide an overview of each board's approach to the problem of sexual misconduct. We asked each board to describe their process for handling complaints of sexual misconduct, including whether specific statutory language is provided. We asked if the boards were experiencing an increasing number of complaints; who filed the complaints; how they investigated allegations of misconduct; and what typical actions were taken. Finally, we requested quantitative data on the number and dispositions of complaints in 1992 and 1993.

We received responses from 34 (52%) boards, including 3 that dealt exclusively with osteopathic physicians. Of these 34 boards, 13 (38%) had statutory language dealing specifically with sexual misconduct. All of the statutes placed complaints of sexual misconduct under the general rubric of unprofessional and/or unethical conduct. For the 21 jurisdictions lacking specific statutory language, 3 (14%) had specific definitions pertaining to sexual misconduct in their administrative rules.

The statutes that contained a definition of sexual misconduct focus on the violation of the physician-patient relationship. For example, the South Dakota statute (South Dakota 1993) states:

> The term unprofessional or dishonorable conduct as used in this chapter includes, but is not limited to:
>
> > (19) The exercise of influence within the physician-patient relationship for the purposes of engaging a patient in sexual activity, and for the purposes of this statute, the patient is presumed incapable of giving free, full and informed consent to sexual activity with the physician.

Or, as defined by the Florida Board of Osteopathic Medicine (Florida 1993):

> The osteopathic physician-patient relationship is founded on mutual trust. Sexual misconduct in the practice of osteopathic medicine means

violation of the osteopathic physician-patient relationship through which the osteopathic physician uses the relationship to induce or attempt to induce the patient to engage, or to engage or attempt to engage the patient, in sexual activity outside the scope of the practice or the scope of generally accepted examination or treatment of the patient. Sexual misconduct in the practice of osteopathic medicine is prohibited.

Or, as defined by the Delaware Board of Medical Examiners (Delaware 1993):

The phrase "dishonorable or unethical conduct likely to deceive, defraud, or harm the public" . . . shall include but not be limited to,

(b) Exploitation of the doctor/patient privilege for personal gain or sexual gratification.

Or, as in Missouri (Missouri 1993):

The board may refuse to issue or renew any certificate of registration or . . . license . . . for one or any combination of causes stated in subsection 2 of this section.

(i) Exercising influence within a physician-patient relationship for purposes of engaging a patient in sexual activity.

Of the 34 reporting boards, 13 (38%) had a formal assessment process that is used during the investigation of a physician for sexual misconduct. Eighteen boards (53%) reported no formal assessment program, whereas three (9%) did not report. Of the 13 with formal assessments, all included psychiatric examination, and 11 (84%) included psychological assessment with the psychiatric examination. Two jurisdictions used a polygraph test as part of their assessments.

We attempted to get an overview of how these boards approached three levels of sexual misconduct: sexual relations with patients, inappropriate touching, and sexually provocative language. Twenty-five (74%) of the boards said that they might use a combination of fine, suspension, and probation for sexual relations with patients; 16 (47%) would use these options for inappropriate touching; and 12 (35%) might use this combination for sexually provocative language.

Finally, we attempted to collect empirical data on the number of sexual misconduct complaints reported in 1992 and 1993. We were interested in the number of complaints filed with each board each year, who filed the complaints, and the board actions in this area, including revocation, suspension, fine, probation, voluntary limitation, and other.

Twenty-seven (82%) boards reported that victims were the primary source of sexual misconduct complaints. Family was listed by 10 (30%) boards as the second most frequent source of complaints, and, in much smaller numbers, the boards listed attorneys and police as the third most likely source of complaints. Very few boards reported that they received reports from professionals.

The survey did not fare well in relation to our request for empirical data on the numbers of complaints received in 1992 and 1993. Fifteen boards (44%) reported either that the statistics were not readily available or they did not have the staff time to complete the survey for 1992, and 13 (38%) could not provide statistics for 1993. This low return rate precludes generalization; however, what was reported was instructive.

Table 5–2 lists the number of complaints reported by the 19 boards that provided data for 1992 and the 21 boards reporting for 1993. The average number of complaints per board increased between these two years. There was a very large range in the number of complaints reported by these boards. In 1993, for example, the 21 reporting boards received between 0 and 131 complaints.

Table 5–3 lists actions taken by the 16 reporting boards in relation to sexual misconduct complaints. There was an average of one revocation per reporting board per reporting year. The "other" category included a variety of actions such as letters of concern and/or warning, reprimand, admonishment, rehabilitation, community service, charity contribution, restriction of practice to males, supervised examinations, and voluntary surrender.

Table 5–2. Total sexual misconduct complaints

	1992	1993
Boards reporting	19	21
Complaints	218	390
Average	11.5	18.6
Range	0–66	0–131

Table 5-3. Board actions

	1992	1993
Boards reporting	16	16
Revocations	17	13
Suspensions	19	20
Probations	19	25
Other	46	45

Discussion

The data presented in this chapter illustrate some initial impressions of how medical boards are currently approaching sexual misconduct cases. The national survey raises many more questions than it answers. The data illustrate the need for further study of what medical boards are actually doing in relation to sexual misconduct cases. Fortunately, a recent study provides much-needed information. In this study of medical board data on sexual misconduct cases reported to Public Citizen's Health Research Group between 1989 and 1994, Dehlendorf and Wolfe (1998) found that rates of disciplinary action for sexual misconduct varied widely among medical boards but that they increased during the study period. On average, 4.1% of disciplinary board orders pertained to sex-related issues, with 72% of these orders resulting in loss or suspension of licenses, compared with 43% for non–sex-related situations.

Physicians disciplined for sexual misconduct were older than the national average physician population and were likely to be involved in direct patient care. Residents were underrepresented in the sample. Similar to the findings in Oregon, Dehlendorf and Wolfe (1998) found that psychiatrists, obstetricians and gynecologists, and family and general practitioners were overrepresented in the disciplined groups.

These authors concluded with a call for increased medical education in the area of professional boundaries and medical ethics and, in addition, an expansion of the laws criminalizing contact between physician and patient.

Another recent study by Morrison and Wickersham (1998) reviewed physicians disciplined in California for an 18-month study period between 1995 and 1997. Sexual misconduct constituted 10% of cases, and 41% of these individuals received what the authors termed *severe discipline,* including revocation, suspension, or letters of reprimand.

To return to our survey, 38% of the reporting boards had specific statutes in relation to sexual misconduct, whereas the rest, like Oregon, handled these cases under statutes addressing unprofessional and unethical conduct. The statutes that were specifically designed for sexual misconduct emphasize the physician-patient relationship and the power that the physician has to "influence" the patient in this relationship (Council on Ethical and Judicial Affairs 1991). This concept of the power to influence, along with the presumption, as expressed in the South Dakota statute, that "the patient is incapable of giving free, full and informed consent" are the same key concepts that are used in these cases in civil and criminal courts (Appelbaum 1990; Strasburger et al. 1991) (see Strasburger, Chapter 2, in this volume).

Most cases in this small sample came to medical board attention from former patients. In Oregon many are now coming to the board in conjunction with the initiation of civil suits. How well is the medical profession doing at policing itself in relation to reports to medical boards? Based on the data presented in this chapter, the answer is not very well. In the national survey, complaints to medical boards originating from other professionals or from ethics committees of professional societies were not listed in the top three sources of complaints to these boards. In the Oregon sample, only a very small number of the complaints came from other providers; one case came from a hospital, whereas none were received from the ethics committees of professional organizations like the medical society or the various subspecialty groups.

More in-depth study is necessary to understand how complaints to medical boards are generated. This is an important issue, because one reading of the data—certainly the popular view—is that very little self-regulation appears to take place in this area. In most situations, medical boards cannot effectively pursue a complaint against a physician unless the complaint originates from a patient, or a specific patient can be identified who is willing to cooperate with the board's investigation. It is possible that other professionals, such as psychotherapists, are involved in a number of the complaints that originate from former patients.

Furthermore, many patients will not permit their physician or therapist to identify them in a specific complaint to a medical board. We all know of situations in which the treating physician is caught between the conflicting mandates of a reporting statute and a privilege statute. This confusing situation requires the physician to choose between opposing courses of action. In such situations most physicians will honor their patient's wishes and respect the preservation of the physician-patient privilege and confidentiality.

How do boards handle the complaints that they do receive? Again we are hampered by the limitations of the data. The best information available is from the study by Dehlendorf and Wolfe (1998). This study makes it clear that the numbers of disciplinary actions per year both varied widely among boards and were also, on average, not very large for a problem with a relatively large prevalence within the physician community (Committee on Physician Sexual Misconduct 1992; Gartrell et al. 1986).

The Oregon data demonstrate that the physicians involved in these complaints were overwhelmingly male, mostly middle-aged (but ranging widely in age from 33 to 83 years), and with an average of 25 years in practice.

The nature of the complaint predicted the outcome. In general, physicians involved with the board because of complaints of inappropriate examination remained in practice, with the large majority of these cases being settled at the Investigative Committee level. In sharp contrast, 74% of the cases involving an accusation of sexual relations with patients were handled by the full board, resulting in almost 50% of these physicians losing or giving up their Oregon licenses.

Complaints involving inappropriate examination are extremely important because they are the most frequent sexual complaints made to the board. Obviously, this is an area where misunderstanding between physician and patient can occur and where physicians should reexamine how they approach patients in relation to breast and pelvic examinations. Extensive use of chaperons and greater patient education should be carefully considered by physicians.

Complaints in this area may also signal more serious problems. Fifty-four percent of the sample had prior complaints made to the board; of those with complaints, 41% (15 physicians) had prior complaints of a sexual nature—mostly complaints related to inappropriate examination. Second complaints in this area should be a signal for more extensive investigation of the situation in the physician's practice and for more assertive intervention by the board.

The board demonstrated a very different pattern of dispositions in relation to cases involving sexual relations with patients. There was a clear difference in disposition between psychiatric and nonpsychiatric physicians. Fifty percent of psychiatrists, compared with 18% of non-psychiatric physicians, no longer had Oregon licenses. It may appear that the board is holding psychiatrists to a higher standard, which may be quite appropriate given the nature of psychiatric practice. Unfortunately, this apparent difference might more accurately mean that psychiatrists give up their licenses more easily and then enter practice as unlicensed psychotherapists.

Physicians with suspected paraphilia represent a small but significant group. The paraphilias are chronic conditions that require expert diagnosis and treatment and are generally of uncertain prognosis. There will be physicians who have various forms of paraphilia. It is important for boards to be aware of this fact and to have the sophistication to differentiate such conditions from other types of sexual misconduct.

Medical boards have been highly successful in developing evaluation and treatment programs for physicians with various forms of substance abuse (Shore 1980; Talbott et al. 1987). In the early 1970s the American Medical Association focused its attention on the development of programs for "impaired physicians": those with mental illness and substance abuse (Council on Mental Health 1973). From that time to the present, medical boards have made great progress, and many have developed sophisticated programs in the diagnosis and treatment of physicians with substance abuse.

This is obviously not the case in relation to the issue of sexual misconduct. Our survey data revealed that only 38% of the boards responding to the survey had formal assessment programs. Although there were no questions on the survey regarding the existence of formal rehabilitation and treatment programs analogous to programs for treating substance abuse, we believe that we would have found that few boards have developed such programs.

In conclusion, we again recognize the central place that medical boards occupy in the life of the physician. These boards have dual responsibilities: they must protect the public from unprofessional, unethical, and poorly informed actions by physicians; but at the same time medical boards have many responsibilities to physicians. These include the provision of rehabilitation programs for physicians who have deviated from acceptable medical practice when rehabilitation does not compromise patient safety. It appears that there is now sufficient information for medical boards to develop evaluation and rehabilitation programs in relation to sexual misconduct (see Gabbard, Chapter 9; and Abel and Osborn, Chapter 10, in this volume). If medical boards pursue this area with the energy and determination that some boards pursued the treatment of substance abuse, both patients and physicians and the integrity of the practice of medicine will be vastly improved.

References

Appelbaum PS: Statutes regulating patient-therapist sex. Hospital and Community Psychiatry 41:15–16, 1990

Committee on Physician Sexual Misconduct: Crossing the Boundaries. The Report of the Committee on Physician Sexual Misconduct. Vancouver, College of Physicians and Surgeons of British Columbia, November 1992

Council on Ethical and Judicial Affairs, American Medical Association: Sexual misconduct in the practice of medicine. JAMA 266:2741–2745, 1991

Council on Mental Health: The sick physician. Impairment by psychiatric disorders, including alcoholism and drug dependence. JAMA 223:684–687, 1973

Dehlendorf CE, Wolfe SM: Physicians disciplined for sex-related offenses. JAMA 279:1883–1888, 1998

Delaware: Del Code Ann tit 24, 1731 (b), 1993

Enbom JA, Thomas CD: Evaluation of sexual misconduct complaints: the Oregon Board of Medical Examiners, 1991 to 1995. Am J Obstet Gynecol 176:1340–1348, 1997

Florida: Fla Stat 459.0141, 1993

Gartrell N, Herman J, Olarte S, et al: Psychiatrist-patient sexual contact: results of a national survey, I: prevalence. Am J Psychiatry 143:1126–1131, 1986

Missouri: Mo Rev Stat 334.100, 1993

Morrison J, Wickersham P: Physicians disciplined by a state medical board. JAMA 279:1889–1893, 1998

Oregon: Oregon Revised Statutes, Chapter 677, 1993

Shore JH: Psychiatric consultation to the Oregon Board of Medical Examiners. Federation Bulletin 67:305–309, 1980

South Dakota: SD Codified Laws Ann Statutes 36–4–30 (19), 1993

Strasburger LH, Jorgenson L, Randles R: Criminalization of psychotherapist-patient sex. Am J Psychiatry 148:859–863, 1991

Talbott GD, Gallegos KV, Wilson PO, Porter TL: The Medical Association of Georgia's Impaired Physicians Program—review of the first 1000 physicians: analysis of specialty. JAMA 257:2927–2930, 1987

Willamette Week, Portland, Oregon 1994

6

SEXUAL MISCONDUCT
The Canadian Experience

Gail Erlick Robinson, M.D., F.R.C.P.C.

In 1990, a case came before the Discipline Committee of the College of Physicians and Surgeons of Ontario (CPSO) in which a physician, not trained as a psychiatrist, had practiced a psychotherapy technique he called "pelvic bonding." The patient had been told to press her face into the male physician's genital area (the patient and the doctor made opposing statements regarding whether or not the physician was wearing his pants at the time). This technique was supposed to remind the patient of the type of security that she, as a child, would have experienced while hugging her father. At that time, the practice of the CPSO was to ask for comments only from another individual who practiced the same type of therapy. No other physicians in the community were involved with this technique, and the handful of lay people who practiced this so-called therapy refused to testify that there was anything wrong with "pelvic bonding." The doctor was therefore exonerated.

When the story was published in the newspapers, the public reacted with an uproar. Although the physicians on the Discipline Committee may have been blinded by the doctor's rationalization that this was "therapy," the public was quick to detect that this explanation was merely an attempt to cover up a form of sexual abuse by a physician. This public embarrassment, in addition to other patient complaints and submissions by such groups as the Metro Toronto Action Committee on Public Violence Against Women and Children (METRAC), resulted in the establishment by the CPSO of the Task Force on Sexual Abuse of Patients by Physicians. It was this task force that led to substantive changes in the understanding of professional sexual misconduct in Canada.

The Canadian System

Each physician in Canada obtains a license to practice from the governing body of his or her particular province, usually called the college of physicians and surgeons. Complaints against a physician are reported to the appropriate governing body. A committee then investigates to determine whether the physician should be subjected to a disciplinary hearing. In Ontario, these hearings take place before a panel of 4 or 5 persons, including at least one lay member. A lawyer for the college acts as prosecutor, and the doctor is defended by his or her own lawyer. Rules of evidence apply. Members found guilty by their colleges may receive penalties ranging from a reprimand to revocation of their license to practice. In addition, most offenders will have their name and the details of their offense published in public college reports. The professional organizations in Canada, such as the Canadian Psychiatric Association, do not investigate or prosecute complaints. Complainants, therefore, do not deal with ethics committees, whose only power is to eject a member from the organization, but rather with the licensing body that can control the member's ability to practice. There is no legislation in Canada defining sexual relations between a health care professional and a patient as a criminal act.

In 1989, the Canadian Psychiatric Association published a position paper on sexual exploitation of patients (Sreenivasan 1989). This paper specified that the "ethical psychiatrist will scrupulously avoid using this relationship to gratify his or her emotional, financial and sexual needs." It noted that, as the idealization and erotic valuation of the therapist is common, psychiatrists may be considered more culpable than other physicians if they engage in sexual activity with a patient. Eroticizing the physician-patient relationship was deemed to be unacceptable under any circumstances, with termination of the therapy, in itself, not being a justification for sexualizing the relationship. The physician was held responsible for resisting advances made by a patient. The statement emphasized the power differential in the physician-patient relationship and noted that they can never be seen as similar to consenting adults. Despite these clear and cogent statements, there was little response from the medical community or the public until the Ontario Task Force was established.

Canadian Prevalence and Beliefs

Public Surveys

Only a few studies examine the prevalence of sexual misconduct by physicians. Two studies examining patients' experiences have been carried out in Canada. In 1991, the Canada Health Monitor—a semiannual national telephone survey of Canadians on matters pertaining to health policy, health promotion, health status, utilization of services, and related matters—studied 549 women 15 years of age and older (Berger and Staisey 1991). Seven percent of these women stated that, during an examination or a consultation, the doctor had watched her dress or undress; made sexual comments about her body or underclothes; made comments about the patient that were sexually demeaning; criticized the patient for her preference in a sexual partner; or made comments about the patient's potential sexual performance. Two percent of the patients stated that they had been involved in actual sexual contact or activity, including kissing, genital-to-genital contact or oral-to-genital contact, or there was touching of genitals or another sexualized body part for purposes other than an appropriate examination. Respondents that answered yes were more likely to be between 25 and 44 years of age and university graduates.

The College of Physicians and Surgeons of British Columbia (CPSBC) also mailed a survey to 6,000 women and 2,000 men chosen at random (Sheps and Schechter 1992). Thirty-five percent of those who received the package responded (35% of women and 18% of men). Of these, 74% stated that a doctor should not ask a patient for a date. The majority believed that a doctor counseling a person for emotional problems should not have sexual contact with that patient during treatment (97%) or after termination of therapy (72%). However, patients were less certain about proper conduct between a former patient and a physician who had been the individual's family doctor for a few years; 40% believed sexual contact was acceptable and 40% unacceptable. Seventy-two percent felt that doctors should not have sexual contact with former patients whom they have counseled for emotional problems. Only 7% of respondents thought that it was acceptable for the only doctor in a small town to have sexual contact with a patient, but 9% indicated they were not sure. Although 4% of the public respondents indicated that the doctor had touched their private body parts for what seemed to be a sexual reason, fewer than 1% of respondents stated that the examining doctor had had sex with them. Fifteen patients (0.7%) reported being asked for a date by a former doctor while seven of the respondents (0.3%) indicated that they had had sexual activity with a doctor after termination of treatment. Of those who had had sexual contact with a physician, 77% indicated they did not report the event.

Professional Surveys

Lamont and Woodward (1994) had a 78% response rate to a survey mailed to all 792 members of the Society of Obstetricians and Gynaecologists of Canada (approximately half of all obstetrician/gynecologists in Canada). The study used the three levels of abuse (sexual impropriety, sexual transgression, and sexual violation) as defined by the CPSO (see Response, below). Three percent of the male respondents and 1% of the female respondents reported sexual involvement with a patient. Ten percent of the respondents indicated that they knew about another obstetrician/gynecologist who, at some time, had been sexually involved with a patient. Seventy-four percent of the respondents supported revocation of the offender's license in cases of sexual violation and 57% in cases of sexual transgression. For cases of sexual impropriety, 33% stated the sentence should involve a reprimand and a fine and 28% believed in rehabilitation without the loss of license. Female obstetrician/gynecologists supported stronger sanctions against sexual transgression and sexual violation than did the men. Whereas 97% of respondents indicated that sexual involvement with current patients is never therapeutic, there were marked differences regarding the propriety of sexual relationships with former patients. Eleven percent of obstetrician/gynecologists felt that no time period was required before beginning to see a former patient socially as long as the professional relationship had been publicly terminated. Another 42% felt that it was proper to begin a relationship within the first year after the termination of a professional relationship. Eleven percent stated that the physician should wait for over a year, and only 14% felt that such a relationship should never occur.

In 1991, the CPSBC conducted surveys of physicians' attitudes to sexual misconduct (Sheps and Schechter 1992). All physicians currently practicing in the province of British Columbia were surveyed, with the exception of those doing primarily laboratory work. A total of 6,245 physicians were sent questionnaires requesting demographic information and knowledge and attitudes concerning a variety of patient contacts. One-third of the sample also received a section inquiring about the individual's actual practices, and an additional third were asked about knowledge of colleagues in his or her specialty who had engaged in the practice in question. Two mailings produced a total response rate of 72% (71% of men and 75% of women).

Eighty-six percent of physicians felt it was unacceptable to ask a patient for a date, whereas 80% disagreed with the statement that there may be some circumstances in which it is acceptable for a physician to have sexual contact with an individual who is his or her patient. Fifty-one percent of physicians (61% of psychiatrists) thought that sexual contact should never occur between a physician and a patient who had been in psychotherapy. About half of the physicians believed it was unacceptable to have sexual contact with a patient whom the physician had seen only once or twice for a "minor" problem. In addition, 62% of physicians disagreed with the statement that it might be acceptable for a physician who is the only doctor in a small town to have sexual contact with a patient.

Of the 1,447 physicians who responded to the questionnaire about their personal practices, 50 (4%) reported that they had had sexual contact with a person who was their patient at the time. Approximately two-thirds of these physicians were involved with one patient, and 24% with two. Ninety-six physicians (7% of the respondents; 84 men [8%] and 12 women [4%]) reported that they had had sexual contact with someone who is a former patient. Posttermination contacts had occurred within 1 month of termination in 23% of cases, within 6 months of termination in 49% of cases, and within 1 year of termination in 71% of cases.

Sixty-three percent of psychiatrists and 21% of physicians had seen patients who had told them of having sexual contact with a previous physician. Twelve percent of respondents indicated that they knew someone who had dated a current patient, whereas 13% knew of a colleague who had had sexual contact with a patient. Psychiatrists (61%) and obstetrician/gynecologists (32%) were far more likely to respond yes to this question. Twenty-one percent of physicians knew of colleagues who had been sexually involved with former patients, almost 80% of these contacts having occurred within 12 months of the termination of the relationship.

Trainee Surveys

A survey of all 535 psychiatric residents in the 16 different programs across Canada (Carr et al. 1991) asked about the education they had received concerning patient-therapist sexual contact. Of the 59% who responded, 21% had had no education concerning patient-therapist sex, 33% had had very little, and only 9% stated that they had had thorough teaching on this topic. Eighteen percent of the respondents believed that patient-therapist sex is permissible after termination of therapy, whereas 81% believed that it is always unethical. Only one resident admitted to having had sexual contact with a patient. The CPSBC, with the cooperation of the Professional Association of Residents and Interns of British Columbia, distributed a questionnaire to residents, interns, and other trainees in all medical specialties in early 1992 (College of Physicians and Surgeons of British Columbia 1992). The response rate was 20%. Ninety-five percent of the respondents said it was not acceptable for a physician to engage in sexual activity with a current patient. When asked the same question with respect to a former patient, 23% said it would not be acceptable, 37% said it would be acceptable, and 38% were uncertain. Thirty-three percent of the trainees said they had not received enough formal or informal training about boundaries, whereas 52% believed that they had received adequate training. In light of the uncertainty about the acceptability of posttermination relationships, one wonders whether this training was in fact adequate.

Ontario

The Ontario Task Force on Sexual Abuse of Patients

The five-member Ontario Task Force on Sexual Abuse of Patients, chaired by an attorney, included two physicians and two nonphysicians. Its mandate was to recommend improvements to college policies and procedures related to sexual abuse complaints; changes to relevant legislation and legal practices; guidelines for doctors with patients and former patients; and educational initiatives for doctors and the public.

Process. The task force, aided by an advisory committee, studied the literature on professional sexual misconduct. In addition, they traveled throughout the province, holding public hearings in a number of cities. A toll-free number also provided an opportunity for patients to anonymously report experiences they had had with physicians. The response was overwhelming. Over 7 months, the task force heard 303 detailed reports of sexual abuse by physicians and others in a position of trust (61 in public or private hearings, 203 through telephone calls, and 39 through letters). The types of abuse included rape and violations of breasts or genitals; representing sex as part of treatment; or the development of personal sexual relationships that disregarded the interests of the patient in order to meet the needs of the physician. They concluded that the college had been doing a poor job of detecting, investigating, and hearing complaints of sexual misconduct on the part of practitioners.

Recommendations. The final report of the task force (College of Physicians and Surgeons of Ontario 1991) made 60 recommendations covering such areas as improved treatment for sexual abuse survivors;

changes in philosophy by the CPSO; changes in education for physicians, the public, and the college; the establishment of guidelines for
doctors; and changes, both inside and outside the college, in the legal
system and the management of survivors. The task force recommended
a zero tolerance standard. This standard establishes that sexual abuse of
patients by physicians is never acceptable and must not be tolerated in
our society. It recognizes the seriousness and extent of injury caused by
such abuse, the risk of harm posed by abusers, and the need for realistic
and effective standards of rehabilitation. Practically speaking, the concept implies that suspected sexual abuse by physicians should be reported and investigated rigorously. It involves a commitment to work
toward the development of a complaints and discipline process at the
CPSO that is both fair and seen to be fair by both patient and doctor. It
also acknowledges that sexual abuse by physicians receives implicit
support in society by judges who do not recognize the seriousness or
nature of sexual abuse involving a breach of trust, the tendency by
many people to disbelieve victims or to deny that such abuse could be
happening, or by the insensitivity of the systems previously in place at
the CPSO that often failed to recognize and adjust for the many obstacles that could prevent a survivor from coming forward. It also emphasizes the importance of educating doctors and the public about
appropriate attitudes, behavior, and treatment boundaries so that abuse
cannot occur out of ignorance. At the same time, zero tolerance does
not mean a lack of support for touch as a crucial healing part of the
practice of medicine when that touch is caring and nurturing rather
than sexual.

The concept of zero tolerance does not mean that doctors convicted
of any type of sexual abuse should automatically lose their licenses.
Two levels of abuse were delineated:

1. *Sexual impropriety:* Any behavior, gestures or expressions that
   are seductive or sexually demeaning to a patient; inappropriate
   procedures such as deliberately watching a patient dress or undress; examination or touching of genitals without the use of
   gloves; inappropriate comments about or to the patient, including sexual comments about a patient's body; initiation by the
   physician of conversation about the sexual problems, prefer-
   ences, or fantasies of the physician; or kissing of a sexual nature.

2. *Sexual violation:* Physician-patient sex, whether initiated by the patient or not, or engaging in any conduct with a patient that is sexual or may be reasonably interpreted as sexual.

The penalties proposed for sexual impropriety would range from a reprimand to temporary suspension of license. The penalty proposed for sexual violation was a mandatory revocation of license for a minimum of 5 years and a fine up to Can$20,000.

The report also set out guidelines concerning involvement with former patients. It was recommended that there be a 2-year time lapse after the last professional contact before sexual involvement is appropriate. In cases where the doctor-patient relationship was primarily for psychotherapy, it recommended a lifetime prohibition on sexual involvement after professional contact due to the powerful, lasting nature of transference, the power imbalance it creates, and the fact that patients often return for further therapy several times over many years. The task force further recommended mandatory reporting by physicians of physician sexual abuse, changes in the complaints and discipline process, and financial compensation to abused patients.

Response. The reaction from the profession was enormous and not always positive. Many physicians felt that the public would see them all as potential abusers and lose their trust in physicians. In addition, they feared that discipline hearings would be slanted so much in favor of the complainants that the doctors would be unable to get a fair trial. Despite these concerns, the college affirmed the principle of zero tolerance and forged ahead in establishing new procedures and rules for the investigation and disciplining of such complaints.

The CPSO defined three levels of sexual abuse of patients:

1. *Sexual impropriety:* Any behavior such as gestures and expressions that are sexually demeaning to a patient or that demonstrate a lack of respect for the patient's privacy;
2. *Sexual transgression:* Any inappropriate touching of a patient, short of sexual violation, that is of a sexual nature;
3. *Sexual violation:* Sex between a physician and a patient, regardless of who initiated it, including, but not limited to, sexual inter-

course, genital-to-genital contact, oral-genital contact, oral-anal contact, and genital-anal contact.

The college started using expert witnesses in hearings of cases of sexual misconduct to help the Discipline Committee understand such issues as why a patient had returned to an offending physician or had taken a long time to report an offense. The prosecutors for the college were able to frame multiple allegations into a specific charge instead of having to address each complaint individually, thus making it easier for complainants to come forward, as well as making it more difficult for individual complaints to be attributed to vengeance or an emotional disorder on the part of the patient.

In 1990, the year of the establishment of the task force, of the 43 sexual abuse investigations commenced, only 14 cases involving three doctors were referred to discipline. Two doctors were found guilty of sexual abuse, whereas the charges against one doctor were withdrawn. In no cases were licenses revoked. In 1993, 127 sexual abuse investigations commenced. The complaints usually involved inappropriate draping, remaining in the room while a patient was preparing for an examination, or making inappropriate remarks. Fifty-nine cases, involving 16 doctors, were referred to discipline. Nine doctors were found guilty of sexual abuse; two were found not guilty; two charges were withdrawn; two cases were dismissed; and one was adjourned. Of the eight revocations of license that year, seven were for sexual abuse (College of Physicians and Surgeons of Ontario 1994).

The task force also stimulated the establishment of programs from the undergraduate to continuing education level concerning physician-patient relationships and sexual misconduct. It also resulted in changes to the Regulated Health Professions Act in Ontario.

Regulated Health Professions Act

The Regulated Health Professions Act (RHPA) of Ontario (1991) governs the professional behavior of 22 different health professions, including physicians, nurses, occupational therapists, pharmacists, and dentists. The final report of the CPSO Task Force on Sexual Abuse of Patients (College of Physicians and Surgeons of Ontario 1991) led to the introduction of Bill 100, an amendment to the RHPA (Ontario

1993) that contains provisions specific to sexual abuse. This bill has underlined the fact that sexual abuse of patients by professionals is not limited to physicians. There are five major components to the sexual abuse amendments: 1) the definition of sexual abuse; 2) a requirement that each professional governing body (college) develop measures to prevent and eradicate sexual abuse by its members; 3) establishment of mandatory reporting of sexual abuse by members; 4) changes to the discipline system to more effectively and sensitively deal with sexual abuse allegations; and 5) establishment of a program to provide funding for therapy and counseling for those who have been sexually abused by practitioners.

Definition.   "Sexual abuse" of a patient by a member of one of the regulated health professions means (Ontario 1993):

   a. sexual intercourse or other forms of physical sexual relations between the member and the patient;
   b. touching of a sexual nature of the patient by the member or;
   c. behavior or remarks of a sexual nature by the member toward the patient.

   Touching, behavior, and remarks of a clinical nature appropriate to the service provided do not constitute sexual abuse. The change from what was previously called "sexual impropriety" to the use of the term "sexual abuse" was made to underline the seriousness of the act. As written in the act, treatment by practitioners of their spouses or lovers would fall within the definition of sexual abuse. The section fails to define when a practitioner and patient relationship has ended and does not address the issue of posttermination relationships.

Measures to prevent and deal with sexual abuse.   Each college is required to clarify its position on sexual abuse and establish a patient relations program to develop measures to prevent or deal with the sexual abuse of patients. Current complaints and discipline processes must be reviewed and guidelines established concerning professional behavior and appropriate conduct with patients.
   Education of trainees and continuing medical education of members are also stressed. Educational programs must cover such areas as what

constitutes sexual abuse; the consequences of sexual abuse; appropriate professional boundaries; and the handling of disclosure by patients of sexual abuse by prior practitioners.

All who deal with abused patients or who investigate or hear allegations of sexual abuse are required to have education to sensitize them to the issues and help them to develop appropriate communication skills. In addition, each college must increase the public's awareness of what constitutes sexual abuse and how to handle complaints of abuse.

Mandatory reporting. Bill 100 requires the mandatory reporting of sexually abusive practitioners by other health care professionals who become aware, in their professional capacity, that such abuse has occurred. In the situation in which a patient identifies an alleged abuser, the patient must be informed of his or her right to complain to the appropriate college and be given information on how to do this. If the patient does not wish to report the abuse, the health care professional is required, within 30 days, to send a written report to the appropriate college. This report must include the name of the reporter, the name of the alleged abuser, and details of the alleged abuse. The patient's name is to be included only if the patient consents in writing. Reports that contain the name of the patient will then be handled by the complaints process of the appropriate college. If the patient wishes to remain anonymous, the report is kept in a special private file and does not become part of the regular record of the alleged abuser. Only if the patient later decides to identify herself, or if a second identified complainant comes forward, will any action be taken. If a second complainant comes forward, the original reporter may be approached by the college to see if his patient is now willing to come forward as part of a joint complaint. The aim of this provision is to provide protection against anonymous complaints for an alleged abuser, while at the same time increasing the possibility of detection of repeat offenders.

Any individual or organization who terminates the employment, revokes, suspends, or imposes limitations on the privileges of a member due to behavior related to professional misconduct must file a report within 30 days. Reporters of suspected sexual misconduct are granted immunity from a civil lawsuit or retaliation in the same way as those who report, in good faith, suspected child abuse.

The most controversial part of this section of Bill 100 is the requirement that a psychotherapist report a health professional who, while in treatment, admits to having sexually abused a patient. This report must also contain an opinion as to whether or not the subject of the report is likely to sexually abuse patients in the future. In addition, immediately upon the cessation of treatment of this individual, a report must be filed indicating that treatment has ceased. The concern of many therapists is that, under these circumstances, abusers will not come forward for treatment.

Changes to the discipline process. Colleges are required to review their discipline processes to make them more effective and more sensitive to the needs of complainants. All colleges now have the power to make interim orders concerning terms, conditions, limitations, or a suspension of an individual's license to practice while under investigation. In the case of sexual abuse involving frank sexual acts, there is a mandatory penalty of both a reprimand and revocation of the license to practice for a period of not less than 5 years, after which an application for reinstatement may be made. Offenders may also be fined up to Can$35,000, as well as being required to reimburse the college for expenses of the investigation and hearing.

In the case of practitioners who have engaged in behavior or remarks of a sexual nature toward a patient, but not sexual touching, Bill 100 offers the possibility of resolving the case by means of an alternate dispute resolution. The practitioner may be required to enter a program to assess his or her knowledge and skills, undergo psychological assessment, or undergo education, therapy, or counseiing. As yet, no governing body in Ontario has established a system for alternate dispute resolution of cases of sexual misconduct.

Therapy program. Bill 100 also requires each college to establish a program to provide funding for therapy and counseling for patients who have been sexually abused by practitioners. The patient has a right to choose his or her own therapist as long as it is not a relative or someone who has previously been a sexual abuser. The maximum amount of funding payable to such a therapist is approximately Can$10,000 over a 5-year period. This is another controversial section of the act. Colleges are required to both finance and oversee the operation of this fund. Financing may have to come from levies on members, mandatory insurance, or the fining of guilty parties. There is very little regulation concerning the type of therapy or counseling received. The patient may receive counseling from someone who is unregulated by any college merely by signing a waiver that he or she understands that this therapist is not subject to professional discipline. This approach runs the risk that patients may end up being treated by untrained therapists who have even less education about the maintenance of boundaries and are not accountable to any governing body.

British Columbia

Process. The College of Physicians and Surgeons of British Columbia (CPSBC) also developed a committee to study the problem of physician sexual misconduct. This nine-member committee (five physicians and four lay members) surveyed the literature (including the final report of the Ontario task force); held public and private hearings; established a toll-free line; surveyed physicians, students and residents, agencies, and the public; met with the medical staffs of 14 hospitals; and surveyed one-doctor communities. Their report, *Crossing the Boundaries,* published in November 1992, made 97 recommendations (College of Physicians and Surgeons of British Columbia 1992).

Recommendations. Sexual misconduct was defined as "exploitation of the physician-patient relationship in a sexual way by the physician's words or actions." The committee recommended that the CPSBC publish a rule that sexual conduct of any kind by a physician with a patient is always unethical. It also recommended that sexual relationships between a physician and a former patient should be presumed to be unethical in any cases in which the physician exploited an imbalance of power present between him or her and the patient as the result of the previous professional relationship; the former patient is under the age of 19 or was when the physician-patient relationship ended; the patient suffers from a disorder likely to impair judgment or hinder independent decision making; or the patient has been in psychotherapy with the physician. If a physician terminates a professional relationship in order to have a sexual relationship with that patient, it should also be considered to be sexual misconduct. The committee proposed that the appropriate penalty for sexual misconduct be a removal of the right to practice medicine. They detailed a number of factors that should be considered in determining the length of the revocation of the license. Mitigating factors would include absence of previous convictions; temporary physical or mental impairment of the physician; inexperience of the physician; evidence of genuine remorse on the part of the physician; and evidence of genuine efforts at rehabilitation. Aggravating factors would include, among others, the degree of exploitation; the vulnerability of the patient; evidence of multiple victims or multiple incidents; and evidence of planned or premeditated activity by the physician. As with the Ontario task force, this committee also made wide-ranging recommendations covering education of professionals and the public and revisions to the complaints process. It further recommended the appointment of a female complaints officer, experienced in dealing with victims of sexual abuse, to handle all complaints of sexual abuse and coordinate educational programs for the college and physicians generally. Although it proposed a statutory obligation for a physician to inform a patient abused by a previous therapist of his or her right to complain to the CPSBC, if the patient would not consent to the filing of a report either with or without his or her name being used, there would be no obligation for the physician to file a third-party report.

Response. Rules made under the Medical Practitioners Act (British Columbia 1994) established a preliminary Review Committee whose responsibility is to consider any complaints that allege or appear to allege sexual misconduct by a member. This committee may direct that the complaint be further investigated, direct that the registrar attempt an informal resolution of the complaint, recommend an appointment of a committee of inquiry, refer the matter to the Ethical Standards and Conduct Review Committee, or direct that no further proceedings be taken. The Ethical Standards and Conduct Review Committee conducts in camera discussions with the complainants and/or member. Generally, its function is to bring the complainant's concern to the attention of the physician under review, educate the physician as to proper practice, and decide if the general application of the issue should be communicated to members of the college to deter other physicians from repeating the conduct that led to the complaint. This committee may make recommendations, set expectations, or issue a warning to the member or may refer the matter to be tried by a committee of inquiry. Sexual misconduct allegations, therefore, may be resolved without ever being referred to the committee of inquiry and the specific offense and offender's name might never be published, even though he pleads guilty. In cases tried by the committee of inquiry, the defendant, if convicted, is found guilty of "infamous behaviour." Penalties may range from a reprimand to the removal of the physician's name from the college register.

Other Provinces

Other provinces and territories have had a variety of responses to the issue of professional sexual misconduct. Alberta developed a Committee on Sexual Exploitation in Professional Relationships (College of Physicians and Surgeons of Alberta 1992), which recommended a two-tiered definition of sexual impropriety and sexual violations. Level one violations would include such things as performing a pelvic examination without gloves; examining breasts, genitals, or anus under false pretenses; kissing and hugging of a sexual nature; and touching or massaging of breasts, genitals, or any sexualized body part for any purpose other than appropriate physical examination or treatment. Sexual violation level 2 would include medical doctor–patient sex, whether initiated by the patient or not, and engaging in any conduct with a patient that is sexual or may be reasonably interpreted as sexual. This committee recommended a penalty of mandatory revocation of license for 5 years and a maximum fine of Can$20,000 for level 1 violations and revocation for 10 years with a maximum fine of Can$50,000 for level 2 violations.

The College of Physicians and Surgeons of Alberta (CPSA), however, decided that boundary violations constitute a continuum that should not be divided into artificial levels of severity. The college endorsed a standard whereby there are no circumstances in which sexual activity between a patient and a doctor is acceptable; it always represents sexual abuse.

The CPSA concluded that relationships with former patients are unethical if there is a potential for the medical doctor to use or exploit trust, knowledge, emotions, or influence derived from a previous professional relationship. Where the medical doctor–patient relationship existed primarily for psychotherapy or family counseling, sexual relationships with the patient are prohibited during the professional relationship and, generally, at any time thereafter. Physicians have an ethical obligation to report conduct by a colleague that might be considered as unbecoming to the profession; failure to report could result in a charge of unbecoming conduct.

A report endorsed by the College of Physicians and Surgeons of Saskatchewan (1992) recommended that the Medical Profession Act be changed to identify sexual abuse and sexual impropriety as physician behavior that is inherently improper. The offense of sexual misconduct is automatically considered more serious if the patient is under age 18; if the physician knew that the patient was particularly vulnerable to sexual overtures; if the physician gained the patient's compliance by the misuse of drugs, hypnotherapy, alcohol, or any other misapplication; or if the physician had been guilty of previous offenses. This report did not specify an automatic minimum offense for conviction. It also did not recommend any single prescribed period of prohibition against relationships with former patients because of the unique circumstances in each case. The committee recommended that physicians should be advised to seek guidance from the college when the propriety of such relationships may be in question. Although this committee did not make recommendations about mandatory reporting, it did note that persons who make reports to the college in good faith should be immune from civil liability for such reporting.

The Special Committee on Sexual Exploitation of Patients by Physicians established by the College of Physicians and Surgeons of New Brunswick (College of Physicians and Surgeons of New Brunswick 1993) also recommended a rule stating that sexual conduct of any kind by a physician with a patient is always unethical and always unacceptable. Consent of the patient should not be a defense to a charge of sexual misconduct. The committee recommended that sexual or romantic relationships with former patients should be viewed as unethical and unacceptable if there is potential for the physician to use or exploit trust, knowledge, emotions, or influence derived from the previous professional relationship. They advised the college to adopt a standard that a physician should not have sexual contact with a former patient until it can be reasonably determined that the patient-physician relationship has been terminated and that the physician is in no position to benefit from a power differential between himself or herself and the former patient. When the patient-physician relationship had been primarily for the purpose of in-depth psychotherapy, the committee recommended that sexual contact with the patient be prohibited during the professional relationship and at any time thereafter. This committee also recommended mandatory third-party reporting of information concerning sexual abuse of a patient by a physician.

The College of Physicians and Surgeons of Manitoba (1992) did not constitute a task force but did issue a statement concerning the definition of sexual exploitation. This was defined as "self-gratifying (for the physician), sexual conversation, dating or suggestions of sexual involvement and/or sexual or romantic contact at any time after the doctor-patient relationship begins and the patient continues to be emotionally dependent on the physician. It could also include a failure on the part of the physician to show reasonable sensitivity for a patient's need for privacy/ territoriality."

The College of Physicians and Surgeons of Prince Edward Island (1993) approved regulations in May 1993 that specifically identified sexual impropriety with a patient as professional misconduct. In response to nationwide media criticism for failing to adequately punish physicians found guilty of sexual misconduct, the Quebec Professional Code was amended in June 1994 (Quebec Legislature 1994). It defined a "derogatory act" as behavior by a physician who, in the course of a professional relationship with a person to whom he is providing services, takes advantage of that relationship to have sexual relations with that person or to make improper gestures or remarks of a sexual nature. The penalty must be, at minimum, a suspension and a fine.

In the other provinces and territories, a practitioner accused of sexual misconduct may be investigated under the general category of unbecoming, improper, unprofessional, or discreditable conduct. Penalties may range from a reprimand to a revocation of license. Some provinces have limited periods for suspension of license, whereas for others there is no limitation. Various restrictions can be placed on the member's practice. Most of the colleges have provisions to impose a fine on a convicted member; moneys obtained in this manner are reimbursed to the provincial health plan. Although many colleges are able to recover costs of the hearing, few have done so. Guidelines to their members about posttermination involvement are often unclear, requiring judgment as to whether or not a power differential still exists. Many provinces do not have any reporting requirements when a physician obtains knowledge about a colleague's sexual misconduct.

Conclusion

Many changes have taken place in the way the Canadian provinces and territories handle the issues of physician sexual misconduct since the embarrassing day in 1990 when the case of "pelvic bonding" hit the press. Perhaps the most impressive changes that have occurred since that time have been those related to physicians' attitudes. From an initial angry and defensive stance, most physicians have come to an increased awareness of the problem of sexual abuse and an increased appreciation of the need for professionalism in their encounters with patients. That is not to say that all the problems have been solved. Many physicians still feel that they have to change previous ways of practice —not for the patient's welfare but rather to guard against an unfair accusation. Some physicians have stated they will no longer do breast or pelvic examinations. The perception by some physicians is that the investigation/discipline process is now weighted in favor of the victim and, once an allegation is made, the doctor will be tried in a "kangaroo court" without any opportunity for defending himself or herself.

Many positive changes have taken place concerning the approach by the colleges. The colleges are more receptive to complaints of physician sexual abuse and most have set up processes to support complainants during the investigation and disciplinary procedures. Discipline committee members have been able to obtain, through the use of expert witnesses, a far more sophisticated understanding of the dynamics and power imbalance involved in patient-therapist sexual relationships and therefore are much less likely to dismiss a case because of assumptions that a patient receiving unwanted advances from a physician would protest loudly, leave the doctor's office immediately, file formal complaints, and certainly never return to the physician.

Education about boundaries in physician-patient relationships has increased exponentially, ranging from the medical student to the most senior level. For example, at the University of Toronto, first-year medical students now receive seminars about sexual misconduct and sexual harassment. In addition, the Faculty of Medicine at the University of Toronto has begun offering a faculty development course designed to educate all directors of postgraduate education about these issues. Teaching about sexual misconduct is now being incorporated into all residency training programs.

Problems remain, however. Although the Canadian Psychiatric Association has stated that termination of a therapeutic relationship in itself is no justification for sexualizing the relationship (Sreenivasan 1989), it has not yet come out with a clear statement such as that of the American Psychiatric Association that sexual involvement with one's former patient is always unethical (American Psychiatric Association 1998). Few colleges have established clear guidelines concerning sexual relationships with former patients. The CPSBC recommendation, for example, seems to imply that there may indeed be some circumstances under which a professional relationship can be terminated to begin a personal relationship. Furthermore, there is no obligation for a college that finds a member guilty of sexual misconduct to report this finding directly to the other colleges. Most colleges report convicted offenders to the Federation of Medical Licensing Authorities. Although the assumption has been that this body will inform all the other colleges, there have been embarrassing instances in which a member convicted by one college has moved to another province and begun to practice. The federation has undertaken to be more diligent in its notification. Although many colleges report convictions to the U.S. National Practitioner Data Bank, there is no automatic check with this bank before granting a license to practice.

Perhaps the most frustrating situation in Canada is that there is no control over who is allowed to practice "psychotherapy." Untrained, "alternative," or lay therapists have no governing body or provincial regulators to oversee their behavior or punish unethical activities. Also, physicians or other health care professionals whose licenses are revoked fall out of the control of any college and no longer have anyone monitoring their behavior. Such individuals can therefore continue carrying on a psychotherapy practice as long as they bill patients directly rather than through a provincial health plan. Although patients may also complain to the police about sexual misconduct, there is a reluctance, commonly seen in victims of sexual abuse, to report to the police and go through the criminal court system. This approach is also complicated by the lack of criminal legislation in Canada concerning sexual relations between a health professional and a patient. In cases where there has been an actual physical sexual assault on the patient, he or she may feel reasonably optimistic about getting a fair hearing in the criminal courts. However, when the patient has been engaged with the physician in a nonviolent sexual relationship, the courts have, until recently, tended to view this as consensual sexual activity between two adults. The courts have also tended to minimize the offense if only one complainant has come forward. There have therefore been some frustrating instances in which a college has revoked the license of a practitioner but, on appeal to the provincial court, the revocation has been reduced to a brief suspension. Although the only way to control these unlicensed practitioners is through provincial or federal legislation, neither level of government has chosen to act on this.

In addition, although many governing bodies have recommended or instituted third-party reporting, there is a concern among physicians that this will interfere with the reporter's relationship with the patient and also may deny natural justice to the accused who may unknowingly have an anonymous complaint on a secret record. The requirement in Ontario to report health professionals who reveal during psychotherapy that they have been abusers can only serve to dissuade abusers from seeking help and, thereby, perpetuate rather than eliminate the problem.

Professional sexual misconduct has now become a topic of major interest for both the public and the professions. It remains to be seen whether the heightened awareness and education concerning professional sexual misconduct will lead to a marked decrease in the incidence of sexual misconduct.

References

American Psychiatric Association: Principles of Medical Ethics With Annotations Especially Applicable to Psychiatry. Washington, DC, American Psychiatric Association, 1998

Berger E, Staisey W: Initial assessment of a survey of Ontario women regarding sexual harassment and abuse by Ontario physicians. Canada Health Monitor, October 27, 1991, pp 1–4

British Columbia: Medical Practitioners Act, ch. 254. Consolidated October 1, 1994

Carr ML, Robinson GE, Stewart DE, et al: A survey of Canadian psychiatric residents regarding resident-educator sexual contact. Am J Psychiatry 148(2):216–220, 1991

College of Physicians and Surgeons of Alberta: Doctor/Patient Sexual Involvement. Policy Paper and Future Initiatives. Edmonton, College of Physicians and Surgeons of Alberta, 1992

College of Physicians and Surgeons of British Columbia: Crossing the Boundaries. The Report of the Committee on Physician Sexual Misconduct. Vancouver, College of Physicians and Surgeons of British Columbia, 1992

College of Physicians and Surgeons of Manitoba: Report on sexuality and the doctor/patient relationship. Winnipeg, College of Physicians and Surgeons of Manitoba, 1992

College of Physicians and Surgeons of New Brunswick: First, Do No Harm. The Report of the Special Committee on Sexual Exploitation of Patients by Physicians. Rothesay, College of Physicians and Surgeons of New Brunswick, 1993

College of Physicians and Surgeons of Ontario: Final Report of the Task Force on Sexual Abuse of Patients. Toronto, College of Physicians and Surgeons of Ontario, 1991

College of Physicians and Surgeons of Ontario: Members Dialogue. September 10–11, 1994. Toronto, College of Physicians and Surgeons of Ontario, 1994

College of Physicians and Surgeons of Prince Edward Island: Regulations Approved by Council. Charlottetown, College of Physicians and Surgeons of Prince Edward Island, May 1993

College of Physicians and Surgeons of Saskatchewan: Report to the Board of the Saskatchewan Medical Association and the Council of the College of Physicians and Surgeons from the Joint Committee re Sexual Abuse of Patients by Physicians. Saskatoon, College of Physicians and Surgeons of Saskatchewan, 1992

Lamont JA, Woodward C: Patient-physician sexual involvement: a Canadian survey of obstetrician-gynecologists. Can Med Assoc J 150(9):1433–1439, 1994

Ontario: Regulated Health Professions Act. SO 1991, C18, 1991

Ontario: Regulated Health Professions Amendment Act. SO 1993, C37, 1993

Quebec Legislature: Act Amending the Professional Code and Other Acts Respecting the Professions, June 1994

Sheps SB, Schechter MT: Attitudes and behaviours in physician-patient relationships: results of surveys of physicians and the public in British Columbia. Vancouver, University of British Columbia, 1992
Sreenivasan U: Sexual exploitation of patients. The position of the Canadian Psychiatric Association. Can J Psychiatry 34:234–235, 1989

SECTION III

Physician Education

7

PREVENTION OF SEXUAL MISCONDUCT AT THE MEDICAL SCHOOL, RESIDENCY, AND PRACTITIONER LEVELS

Jerald Kay, M.D., and Brenda Roman, M.D.

Although the Hippocratic Oath has prohibited physician-patient sexual relations for centuries, and current ethical thought condemns such actions, sexual misconduct by physicians continues to occur at a significant rate. A 1992 survey of 10,000 family practitioners, internists, obstetrician-gynecologists, and surgeons found that 9% of respondents acknowledged sexual contact with patients (Gartrell et al. 1992). Of all practicing gynecologists and otolaryngologists in the Netherlands, 4% of the respondents had had sexual contact with a patient (Wilbers et al. 1992). A survey of psychiatrists in the United States revealed that 7% of male and 3% of female respondents admitted having sexual contact with their own patients (Gartrell et al. 1986). In a 1988 survey of senior psychiatry residents, nearly 1% acknowledged sexual involvement with a patient (Gartrell et al. 1988). Due to the probable hesitancy to respond to such questionnaires, the actual incidence of sexual misconduct by physicians and residents is likely higher. Despite legal sanctions, malpractice suits, and ethical prohibition by professional organizations (American Medical Association 1991; American Psychiatric Association 1993, 1998) and state medical licensure agencies, the problem continues.

Although physicians who engage in sexual contact with patients offer various explanations for their behavior, some "never thought about the physician-patient relationship in any meaningful way until after they were in deep trouble" (Bloom et al. 1991, p. 1370). One may conclude, therefore, that the problem continues, in part, due to a lack of education regarding the traumatic impact that sexual relationships have on patients. In fact, two of the earliest surveys on this subject found that 10% of doctors considered "erotic contact with a patient may be beneficial" (Kardener et al. 1973), and 25% of first-year medical students believed that sexual intercourse with a patient could be appropriate if the doctor was "genuine" and the circumstances were right (Wagner 1972). More recently, 19% of female physicians and 40% of male physicians did not believe that physician-patient sexual misconduct was always harmful to the patient (Gartrell et al. 1992).

The issue of physician sexual misconduct has not been addressed effectively during medical school or residency. Of United States physicians surveyed in 1992, 56% of respondents said sexual conduct had not been addressed in their training and only 3% had participated in a continuing education course focusing on this topic (Gartrell et al. 1992). Over half of Canadian senior psychiatry residents surveyed indicated that they had received little or no education regarding sexual issues between psychiatrists and patients (Blackshaw and Patterson 1992). In short, it appears that medical students, residents, and practitioners have received little instruction in the matter of physician sexual misconduct.

Role of Education as a Basic Approach to Preventing Sexual Misconduct

Since codes of ethics, regulations, and instruction regarding sexual misconduct from national medical organizations, state medical boards, and specialty societies have been readily available, especially very recently, the simple distribution of literature to address this complex issue appears to be rather ineffective. A more organized educational approach, with an appropriate emphasis on the proper physician-patient relationship throughout a physician's education, is indicated. This should begin in the preclinical medical school curriculum so that it is possible to prevent physician sexual misconduct, rather than undertake the more difficult task of rehabilitation of the offender at a later time. Education offers opportunities 1) to learn about the potential problem of sexual misconduct; 2) to shape attitudes about proper professional relationships; 3) to acquire skills to handle the feelings that may be evoked by patients; and 4) to identify the responses that occur within the physician that are independent of the patient and derive from the physician's psychological vulnerability.

There are a number of effective educational approaches to meet these goals, including the use of audiovisual stimulus films, role playing, problem-based learning, case discussions, simulated patients, and clinical supervision. Most importantly, however, this subject matter must be revisited throughout the physician's entire professional career. We will examine the specifics of these educational approaches for each professional developmental stage.

Educating Medical Students About Sexual Misconduct

Instruction in medical ethics has only recently been required in the medical school curriculum. However, in most medical ethics courses, sexual misconduct is not considered a prominent ethical issue and is therefore rarely addressed (Miles et al. 1989; Perkins 1989; Sulmasy et al. 1990). This deficiency is dramatically illustrated in Table 7–1, which provides, from an extensive review of the literature, the suggested topics for comprehensive ethical instruction in the medical student curriculum (Miles et al. 1989). Conspicuous by its absence in the summary table, as well as in the text of the manuscript, is any specific reference to the problem of sexual misconduct.

The entering and graduating classes at Stanford University School of

Table 7–1. Content areas for medical ethics education

Ethical theory and humanities
 Basic bioethical concepts
 Religious theory and medicine
 Humanities
Professional ethos
 Codes of ethics in medicine
 Physician bias about patient's quality of life
 Duty to treat HIV-infected persons
 Compassion
 Rights and duties of doctors
 Determination of death
 Pain control
 Organ donation, requests, selecting recipients
 Innovative technology
 Physicians and cost constraints or economic incentives
Multidisciplinary issues
 Impaired colleagues
 Consultation and team ethics
 Differences with colleagues
 Relations with lawyers, nurses, and reporting agencies
 Use of ethics consultants and committees
Patient autonomy and clinical dilemmas
 Autonomy and personhood
 How patients relate risk to values
 Obtaining consent
 Patients' refusal of recommended treatments
 Truth-telling and withholding information from patients
 Patient privacy and confidentiality
 Evaluation of decision-making capacity
 Proxy consent, informed consent, coerced consent
 Role of families in treatment decisions
 Sexual responsibility

(continued)

Table 7-1.	Content areas for medical ethics education (*continued*)

Patient autonomy and clinical dilemmas (*continued*)

Abortion

Defective newborns

Maternal-fetal conflicts

Rights of children, psychiatric patients, handicapped persons

Artificial insemination, in-vitro fertilization

Care of the dying, comatose, or hopelessly ill

Forgoing life support

Euthanasia

Student physicians

Academic integrity

Revealing student status to patients

Student's feeling of excess entitlement

Disclosure of new information to patients

Role of student physicians

Academic medicine

Authorship

Research ethics

Social issues

Preventive medicine; health and disease concepts

Justice and health care

Legal medicine, forensic medicine, malpractice

Nuclear war

Genetics

Community service

Source. Reprinted from Miles SH, Weiss-Lane L, Bickel J, et al.: "Medical Ethics Education: Coming of Age." *Acad Med* 64:705–714, 1989. Used with permission.

Medicine were surveyed to determine the difference in attitudes between the two groups regarding romantic relationships between physicians and patients (Granich and Mermin 1992). Nearly one-fifth of both entering and graduating students felt it was appropriate for a physician to develop a romantic relationship with a patient. Approximately the same number of both student groups were undecided about the appropriateness of such behavior, and, strikingly, there were no statistically significant differences between the responses of the entering and graduating classes. That no changes in attitudes were demonstrable between these two groups raises serious questions about the education in ethics they receive.

There have always been cynical voices in medical education that have questioned the student's capacity to be influenced in moral matters, preferring instead to conceptualize ethical and moral reasoning as being related to early personality development completed prior to matriculation in medical school. Others have demonstrated that this may not be the case (Self et al. 1992, 1993). Growth in moral reasoning among medical students is predicated on the acquisition of new information within novel contexts. The components of morality in medical student education (Rest 1988) may be conceptualized as 1) recognition of issue (i.e., physician sexual misconduct exists); 2) judgment about what is right (i.e., a physician-patient sexual relationship is never appropriate); 3) priority of moral values over personal values (i.e., even if not in full agreement about the impact on patients, there is student acceptance of established ethical guidelines); and 4) perseverance to implement one's moral intention (i.e., if sexual feelings toward a patient develop, seek appropriate consultation to ensure that the feelings are never acted on, thus maintaining the proper physician-patient relationship).

Since students do not automatically accept that physician-patient sexual relationships are unethical, a key element in any successful instruction must emphasize the enormous psychic harm that occurs to such patients (Feldman-Summers and Jones 1984). Students should be informed that these patients may suffer from complex posttraumatic stress disorder, anxiety and depressive disorders, sexual symptoms, dissociative disorders, and sleep disturbances and are at higher risk for substance abuse, psychiatric hospital admission, and suicide (Bouhoutsos et al. 1983; Feldman-Summers and Jones 1984; Gartrell et al. 1988; Pope and Bouhoutsos 1986). In addition, these patients experience great discomfort in future doctor-patient relationships, which can eventuate in less-than-optimal medical care. Intense feelings of shame, guilt, and mistrust are the rule in such relationships, especially in light of the fact that many women who have been traumatized through physician sexual misconduct were also victims of childhood sexual abuse (Feldman-Summers and Jones 1984; Kluft 1989).

Gartrell et al. (1992) identify several issues that all students should appreciate. Educators must teach that sexual contact between physicians and patients violates the fiduciary nature of the relationship that requires physicians to act in the best interest of their patients. "The therapeutic relationship is balanced on knife edge, the slightest slip leading to dauntingly complex psychological sequelae for patient and physician" (Fisher and Fahy 1992, p. 3). When seeking medical care, patients, regardless of their sophistication, are psychologically and often physically vulnerable and dependent on the physician's medical expertise. During this process, moreover, patients routinely develop feelings of trust and respect for their physicians—feelings that are instrumental in the promotion of a beneficial doctor-patient relationship. Because patients feel gratitude toward their doctors and there is an imbalance of power in the doctor-patient relationship, patients may find it difficult to decline sexual invitations from their physicians. It is always the physician's responsibility to prevent the relationship from developing into a harmful sexual one. In addition, patients generally receive inadequate medical care from physicians with whom they are sexually involved, often because of the diffusion and contamination of roles and the inherent conflicts that arise from such a distorted relationship.

Students should also be informed of the patient groups considered to be at high risk for being lured into unduly familiar relationships (Simon 1992). These include 1) previously well-functioning patients with significant current depression and recent loss of a love relationship; 2) those who were sexually and physically abused in childhood; 3) patients with histories of psychiatric illness, especially those that include suicide attempts, psychiatric hospitalizations, and substance abuse; 4) patients with documented personality disorders, specifically those with borderline, dependent, masochistic, and histrionic features; and 5) patients with marked low self-esteem. However, one must view all patients as potentially vulnerable.

Many medical school curricula contain some instruction on student and physician well-being and impairment. These lectures usually detail the stresses and strains inherent in preparing for a career in medicine as well as those encountered in the actual practice of medicine. Instruction frequently presents the incidence of substance abuse and suicide among practitioners. The need for having one's own physician, and the helpfulness of exercise and planning methods for professional activities are often covered as well. Rarely, however, is mention made of physician vulnerability and the possibility of sexual misconduct. Many faculty members feel reluctant to introduce to students the possibility that some physicians become despondent and frustrated in their practices and turn to their patients to compensate for feelings of loneliness, unworthiness, and incompetency. Similarly, it is rarely noted that marital unhappiness and illness can predispose physicians to sexual misconduct. The examination of these predispositions should be a component of lectures in behavioral science courses on the developmental aspects of work and physicianhood. It is also important that such instruction not be limited to misconduct among male physicians.

Even the most comprehensive didactic instruction will be less effective educationally if there is not an institutional commitment to address such topics as sexual harassment and the overall abuse of medical students by faculty, residents, and staff (Bourgeois et al. 1993; Kay 1990; Sheehan et al. 1990; Silver and Glicken 1990). The strict enforcement of sexual harassment policies and the prohibition of lecture room sexual jokes that demean women establishes an important institutional ethos regarding the seriousness of the power dynamics between men and women physicians, students, and their patients.

Medical school curriculum committees should be charged, as they are in other subject or topic areas, to monitor the instruction about sexual misconduct throughout all four years of the student's education. There should be both horizontal and vertical curricular integration so that this topic is reinforced wherever possible across departmental boundaries. For example, a phase-appropriate education schema might consist of the topics illustrated in Table 7–2.

Instruction about sexual misconduct should not be limited to lectures. Medical ethics is best taught through small group discussion that is case centered with opportunities for role playing and discussion of audiovisual tapes when appropriate. These pedagogical techniques permit the shaping of attitudes and values about the characteristics of proper physician-patient relationships. The ability to discuss sexual misconduct under the leadership and supervision of faculty also establishes the model of promoting consultation with colleagues around sensitive issues in medical practice.

Table 7-2.   Suggested topics for ethical instruction in the medical student curriculum

Year	Course	Topic
I	Behavioral Science & Introduction to Psychiatry	Essentials of the doctor-patient relationship, including transference, countertransference, the illness experience, and the contribution of early development and personality in illness
		Human sexuality
		Physician well-being and impairment
	Introduction to Medical Ethics & Jurisprudence	Ethical and legal aspects of sexual misconduct
II	Medical Interviewing	Recognizing and managing nontherapeutic responses to patients
	Physical Diagnosis	Implications of power dynamics and the need for explicit boundaries
		Limitations of touching patients
		Importance of chaperoning
III/IV	Clerkships	Review and integration of topics covered in years I and II as they relate to supervised patient care experiences in individual clinical departments (internal medicine, surgery, obstetrics-gynecology, psychiatry, etc.)
		Clinical conferences should integrate ethical issues in all patient presentations

Educating Residents About Sexual Misconduct—An Overview

Medical education often involves the revisiting of basic material with increasing sophistication in succeeding phases. Thus the topics to be addressed in residency about physician sexual misconduct are not dramatically different from those described for undergraduate medical education. In many respects, however, the experience of the house officer is different from that of the medical student. The clinical responsibilities of the resident are performed under less intensive supervision. Moreover, the resident's experiences with patients are more in-depth and are likely to cause greater anxiety. Pressures on interns and residents have increased in teaching hospitals because of greater patient acuity, decreased lengths of stay for patients, and larger amounts of required paperwork. Challenging on-call responsibilities may predispose residents to feelings of inadequacy, fatigue, loneliness, depression, and anxiety and a sense of disconnectedness from people. It is not surprising, therefore, that some residents choose to combat these feelings through sexual encounters. These can occur between residents and nurses, medical students, and even patients (Gartrell et al. 1988). Thus, there is greater immediacy in residency training to the issue of sexual misconduct.

Ethical instruction in residency training is not nearly as consistent or structured as in medical school. In addition, it suffers from some of the same narrow conceptualizations regarding appropriate ethical instructional content (Sulmasy et al. 1990). In a recent review of the teaching of medical ethics during residency training, the following ethical skills were deemed the most fundamental for all residents. They should know (Perkins 1989)

- The moral aspects of medical practice—the process of clarifying the patient's versus the doctor's values about treatment
- How to obtain informed consent
- What to do if a patient refuses recommended treatment
- What to do about incompetent patients
- When it is morally justified to withhold information
- When breaching confidentiality is justified
- How to manage patients with poor prognoses
- How to manage medical resources wisely

Although these core skills are admirable and should be mastered by all residents, conspicuous by its absence is knowledge about the boundaries of the helping relationship. An ethics curriculum for residency programs should include general ethical principles, one component of which must be the ethical dimensions and the psychological characteristics of the doctor-patient relationship. Upon this framework can be added issues of informed consent, confidentiality, truth telling, life-sustaining treatment concerns, and allocation of scarce resources.

In general, the success of an ethics program within a clinical department depends heavily on the endorsement of the faculty—in particular, the residency training director and the chair. Because ethics didactics vary significantly from program to program, the personal commitment by the faculty is probably the single most critical aspect in the continuity of instruction. It is also helpful to have specially trained faculty members who teach ethics within the residency program. There are a number of intensive courses and fellowships in medical ethics that prepare clinical faculty members for teaching within their training programs. These opportunities include instruction in patient-centered ethical consultations as well as suggestions about seminar topics and effective teaching methods (Perkins 1989). The use of medical ethicists from other departments and universities who establish regularly scheduled ethics rounds has proved to be effective in some programs. However, issues of sexual misconduct are generally not the focus of such instructional programs and surface only if there has been formally recognized unethical behavior among the housestaff. We regularly give didactics to nonpsychiatric housestaff (primarily internal medicine and family medicine) on boundary issues in clinical practice. It is useful for the residents to read Gabbard and Nadelson's article "Professional Boundaries in the Physician-Patient Relationship" (Gabbard and Nadelson 1995) beforehand. The structure is then set to discuss the concept of boundaries in clinical medicine, focusing initially on sexual boundary violations. Once the residents begin to wrestle with the issue of a relationship with a former patient—even one involving only a one-time physician-patient contact—the stage is set to begin examining the issues of dual relationships, gifts, time and duration of appointments, language, self-disclosure, and physical contact with patients in much greater depth.

Psychiatry Residency Education

Despite the professed attention by the psychiatric establishment to matters of sexual misconduct, surveys of psychiatric resident education on the topic are disquieting. A national survey of all American psychiatric residents in postgraduate year 4 (PGY-IV) revealed that only 12% reported receiving a thorough education within their residency programs about the sexual exploitation of patients (Gartrell et al. 1988). Similarly, a survey of Canadian psychiatric residents revealed that more than 50% of the residents received little or no education on physician sexual misconduct (Carr et al. 1988). A 1989 survey of all United States psychiatry residency training directors found that only 20% specifically included topics on psychiatrist-patient sexual contact, despite 46% of the program directors responding that the topic is "most note-worthy" (Coverdale et al. 1992). In that same survey, 43% of responding chief residents in psychiatry believed that physician-patient sexual contact should be addressed during residency education.

Although Freud emphasized the principle of interpreting, as opposed to acting on, erotic feelings within the treatment relationship (Freud 1915/1958), the psychiatric profession until recently has minimized the issue of sexual misconduct, which may have contributed to continuing misconduct. Another significant impediment to comprehensive instruction in sexual misconduct is the level of discomfort among residents in discussing erotic issues during supervision. In a survey of Canadian psychiatry residents, 85% of respondents indicated that it was normal to experience sexual feelings toward patients, and nearly the same number (79%) thought these feelings should be discussed in supervision. However 45% felt unable to discuss attraction to patients in supervision. They believed that their supervisors actively discouraged discussing these issues, and they feared that they would be evaluated poorly, or they were concerned that raising the topic might be misconstrued by the supervisor as a sexual invitation (Blackshaw and Patterson 1992).

There are striking consequences from not being able to discuss feelings of attraction during the supervisory process; in particular, the resident never experiences the profound meaningfulness of romantic feelings for both the doctor and patient and that such feelings dissipate when the meaning is fully appreciated. In addition, in many programs, the concept of boundaries, particularly boundary violations, is not thoroughly addressed. The therapeutic or professional boundaries include the role of the therapist, the time and place of the appointment, fees and payments for services, gifts, the therapist's clothing, the therapist's use of language, physical contact, and self-disclosure (Gutheil and Gabbard 1993). Violations of these boundaries almost always precede the extreme boundary violation of sexual misconduct.

Certainly not all boundary violations lead to sexual misconduct, and boundary violations do not always constitute malpractice or misconduct. However, civil or criminal juries and state licensing boards increasingly seem to accept that the presence of boundary violations is presumptive evidence that corroborates allegations of sexual misconduct (Gutheil and Gabbard 1993). As recommended by legal experts, if a physician feels that touching a patient is indicated for therapeutic reasons, such interventions should be scrutinized carefully and should be documented to prevent misinterpretation (Gutheil and Gabbard 1993). Residents should be reminded that intended nonsexual touch can be misinterpreted by any patient. For example, a touch that is meant to convey warmth can actually be frightening to some patients. It is helpful for residents to consider the implications of touching a terminal patient being assessed on an oncology service as opposed to touching a long-term psychotherapy patient. In nearly all instances, empathy and warmth can be conveyed through words just as effectively without the potential liability of misinterpretation.

A Psychiatric Residency Curriculum in Sexual Misconduct

The Canadian Psychiatric Association has endorsed residency training guidelines for ethical instruction on physician sexual misconduct (Blackshaw and Patterson 1992). According to these guidelines, any training program should include the following essential components:

- Information on ethical prohibitions on doctor-patient sexual involvement. This information should be disseminated early in the training program.
- Formal review of the scientific literature on sexual exploitation of patients. Particular attention should be given to the elements of

abuse of power, breach of trust, and tendency toward reenactment by patients who have had previous traumatic experiences.

- Introduction to gender-related issues, gender role behavior, and gender role socialization and their contributions toward power imbalances in male-female relationships.

- Supervisory training on sexual issues. Because the supervisory relationship is not therapeutic and is therefore noninterpretive, it is the major learning experience for issues of sexual attraction that arise within the therapist-patient relationship. The resident should be taught that acting on sexual impulses toward a patient is forbidden at all times. However, such feelings should be brought to the supervisor for discussion. Residents should also be taught that these feelings are a component of broader countertransferential reactions that are instructive for every therapist. Supervisors also should convey the preventive importance of seeking consultation when the physician experiences intrusive erotic feelings when working with patients.

One critical area not addressed by the Canadian guidelines is the need for residents to be aware of the civil and criminal statutes regarding doctor-patient sexual intimacy in their state. Without such knowledge, residents will not be able to provide comprehensive treatment to patients who have been victimized by previous professionals, because informing patients of their legal options is a central task in treating these patients. In addition, it would be helpful for all residents to have an appreciation for the current legal issues surrounding sexual misconduct, such as mandatory reporting initiatives, when similar laws are not in force in their own states. The fundamental question of whether it is ever permissible to have an extraprofessional relationship with someone whom you have treated should be a part of every educational program.

Although some residency programs provide intensive short courses, we propose a longitudinal framework for education about physician sexual misconduct (Table 7–3) because it allows revisiting the topic after having new clinical experiences. In PGY-I, instruction should focus on the proper physician-patient relationship, including its fiduciary nature, through an introduction to the central concepts of transference, countertransference, therapeutic neutrality and abstinence. Boundary violations and the specific ethical prohibitions regarding sexual in-

Table 7–3. Topics for residency curriculum on sexual misconduct

Postgraduate year	Topic
I	Physician-patient relationship
	Concept of boundary violations
	Ethical and legal prohibitions about physician-patient sexual involvement
	Discussion of the Exploitation Index
II	Gender issues and power imbalances in male-female relationships
	Effects of psychic trauma
	Patient vulnerabilities
	Physician vulnerabilities
	Further discussion of boundaries and the Exploitation Index
III and IV	Proper management of erotized transferences and countertransference
	Treating the patient who has been sexually exploited by a previous therapist
	State civil and criminal statutes about physician-patient sexual intimacy

Source. Adapted from Roman and Kay 1997.

volvement with patients should be elucidated within the first year of training. All beginning psychiatric trainees should receive and discuss the American Psychiatric Association's (APA's) *Principles of Medical Ethics With Annotations Especially Applicable to Psychiatry* (American Psychiatric Association 1998). In addition, *Resource Document: Legal Sanctions for Mental Health Professional–Patient Sex* (American Psychiatric Association 1993), although not official APA policy, is a highly succinct introduction to all aspects of the topic. Many residency training programs have found that two videotapes produced by the APA Office of Education, entitled *Ethical Concerns About Sexual Involvement Between Psychiatrists and Patients* (American Psychiatric Association 1986) and *Reporting Ethical Concerns About Sexual Involvement With Patients* (American Psychiatric Association 1990), have been effective in small discussion groups with beginning and advanced residents. Both of these videotapes are available through the American Psychiatric Press and are packaged with helpful discussion guides for group leaders. There are many brief clinical vignettes on each of these tapes, so that some may be shown early in training to residents and others later during the advanced years. During PGY-II and PGY-III, didactics should focus on the effects of psychic trauma and introduce the concept of complex posttraumatic stress disorder as a background for appreciating the impact of sexual trauma and the power of traumatic reenactments. There is no finer introduction for residents to these topics than that found in *Trauma and Recovery* by Judith Herman (Herman 1992). In our experience, residents have been universally challenged by this exceptional book.

In addition, the scientific literature on the sexual exploitation of patients should be reviewed, focusing on the abuse of power and the breach of trust in the physician-patient relationship. Issues of boundary violations, particularly their legal implications, need to be explored. As residents learn effective outpatient treatment strategies for their patients, they should be cognizant of the greater likelihood of boundary violations with patients suffering from primitive personality disorders. Specific countertransferences that are common in the treatment of borderline personality disorder, for example, have been described by Gabbard and Wilkinson (1994). These include intense guilt feelings, rescue fantasies, transgression of professional boundaries, helplessness and worthlessness, anxiety and terror, and rage and hatred for the patient. It should also be noted that in an attempt to ward off powerful negative feelings evoked by their patients, inexperienced residents frequently sexualize their responses to such patients as well.

Because most cases of physician sexual misconduct occur between female patients and male physicians, the power imbalances in male-female relationships should be explored through instruction on gender role behavior and gender role socialization.

Senior-level residents should understand the proper management of erotic transferences and countertransferences. We have found that, because residents are generally hesitant to discuss erotic feelings in supervision, a discussion-group format with a senior psychiatrist presenting his or her own clinical material and acknowledging erotic feelings provides a more comfortable atmosphere for residents to discuss such issues. Through discussion and modeling, the residents will be better prepared to handle their own erotic feelings in clinical work and will probably be more likely to seek consultation. Moreover, since 50% of all psychiatrists will at some point during their careers treat a patient who has been sexually involved with a previous therapist, the specific literature on treating such patients should be presented (Kluft 1989; Notman and Nadelson 1994). Patients who have been sexually involved with former clinicians present subsequent therapists with unique clinical issues that must be attended to in the new treatment relationship if it is to be successful (see Notman and Nadelson, Chapter 11, in this volume).

Besides formal courses and grand rounds, some programs have found it useful to conduct mock trials, provide victim-advocate presentations, and have actual perpetrators and victims present their experiences. More commonly, other programs present role-playing scenarios of situations that lead to sexual misconduct (Pope and Bouhoutsos 1986). These include "role trading," in which the therapist becomes the center of the treatment; "sex therapy," in which the patient is presented with the notion that sexual relations between therapist and patient is a helpful treatment technique; "as if," wherein the therapist attributes the patient's positive transference as reality; "Svengali," in which the patient's dependency is exploited; "drugs," in which the use of substances becomes part of the seduction or as a trade for sex; "true love," wherein the physician rationalizes and disavows the professional relationship and its inherent responsibilities; "it just got out of hand," wherein the therapist is unable to address emerging feelings within the treatment relationship; "time out," in which the therapist falsely conceptualizes that the professional relationship is not in force after formal appointment times; and "hold me," in which the therapist takes advantage of the patient's wish for nonsexual contact; this scenario underscores the important concept that in most cases nonsexual contact precedes sexual experiences.

Since research has found that minor boundary violations generally precede physician sexual misconduct, the issues of maintaining boundaries in therapy once again need to be emphasized. Residents must appreciate that if minor boundary violations are employed, a reason must exist, supported by documentation as to why such a boundary crossing was therapeutically indicated (Gutheil and Gabbard 1993). One effec-

tive introduction to the concept of boundary violations is the administration to residents of the Exploitation Index developed by Epstein and
colleagues (Epstein et al. 1992). This 32-item questionnaire covers a
variety of boundary issues such as prescribing medication for family
members, touching patients, deceiving third-party payers, and therapist self-revelation. The Exploitation Index is an exceptionally thorough self-assessment tool that has been validated with high internal
consistency in a systematically sampled population of 532 psychiatrists
(Epstein et al. 1992).

All residents must appreciate the career consequences of sexual misconduct. We have strongly educated about the phenomena of a "slippery slope" and have taught residents that, in many ways, sexual
misconduct is the quickest method of professional suicide. We repeatedly emphasize that only the psychiatrist—and not the patient—has a
professional code that can be violated, and therefore only he or she can
be culpable, liable, and, in some states, criminal. Residents are dis-
abused of the notion that patient-initiated sexual activity is possible
(Gutheil and Gabbard 1993). Residents must understand as well the
justification for criminal statutes aimed at psychiatrists who become
sexually involved with their patients and the fact that there are strong
calls for such statutes in the 36 states that do not yet have them. Residents are informed of the many legal precedents established in sexual
misconduct cases. For example, trainees often believe it is possible to
avoid the ethical-legal consequences of sexual misconduct by marrying
a patient. They are informed that this is not the case (CV NOS DR
1989). Residents are also made aware that the APA has recently published a fact sheet on patient-therapist sexual contact that is available to
the public and clearly warns patients of specific exploitative boundary
violations (American Psychiatric Association 1992).

Finally, it must be emphasized that the most helpful actions in pre-
venting false sexual misconduct allegations are comprehensive diagnoses, well thought-out treatment plans, thorough documentation of all
treatment, and provision of the very best clinical care. Seeking consultation with other colleagues is an integral part of this approach, especially when treating complex patients. Although it is out of fashion
these days to advocate personal psychotherapy for trainees, such an experience frequently provides the resident an additional opportunity to
discuss and understand the importance of strong feelings for patients.

Relationship of Resident-Educator Sex to Physician Sexual Misconduct

Although data are not available to support the theory, we believe that if sexual boundary violations occur in resident-educator relationships, such violations may be more likely to occur subsequently with patients. Certainly the rates of resident-educator sexual relationships are disconcerting, with 4.9% of 548 United States residents in PGY-IV affirming a sexual relationship with a teacher (Gartrell et al. 1988) and 2.5% of Canadian psychiatric residents reporting sexual involvement with their teachers (Carr et al. 1988). Although these findings are considerably below the 13.6%–22% rates of involvement between psychology graduate students and their professors (Glaser and Thorpe 1986; Robinson and Reid 1985), they are nevertheless significant for a number of reasons.

Sexual involvement between a student and teacher, regardless of the student's age, has many parallels to that of sexual relations between therapist and patient. First, the student, like the patient, is in many respects the less powerful member of the dyad. Just as transference feelings are universal between doctor and patient, the teacher also serves as an important transference object for the student. Furthermore, strong feelings of appropriate idealization for teachers are common on the part of students and can also be manipulated. Second, as is the case in nearly all student-teacher relationships, the student is dependent on the educator with respect to performance evaluation. Third, sexual involvement shortchanges the student of an impartial evaluation of progress. Fourth, residents who are sexually involved with their supervisors are likely to have greater difficulty discussing with their supervisors issues of sexual feelings in their own clinical work, thereby depriving the resident of significant professional development regarding comfort in role definition and professional boundaries (Pope 1989).

Educating Nonpsychiatric Residents

Ideally, the concepts proposed as essential knowledge for psychiatry residents should be covered in all medical specialties. As stated previ-

172 PHYSICIAN SEXUAL MISCONDUCT

ously, the problem of physician sexual misconduct is not unique to psychiatry; in fact, in Gartrell's (1992) survey of 10,000 physicians, 11% of family physicians and 10% of obstetrician-gynecologists acknowledged sexual contact with patients—higher rates than those found in surveys of psychiatrists (Gartrell et al. 1986). This finding may be partly due to these adult primary care specialists receiving little if any training on this ethical issue and being unaware of the very powerful nature of the physician-patient relationship. In an article on developing an ethics curriculum for a family practice residency (Levitt et al. 1994), no mention was made about the issue of physician sexual misconduct, despite increased attention to this issue in the media. With a significant incidence of reported physician-patient sexual contact, it is clear that all adult primary care physicians need comprehensive instruction about the problems of physician sexual misconduct. The basic areas outlined for a psychiatry residency curriculum could be easily adapted to other residency curricula. For other specialties, ethical prohibitions on sexual misconduct need to be addressed. In addition, the traumatic impact on patients should be thoroughly explored, as should physician vulnerabilities to sexual misconduct, as minimum curriculum requirements.

Continuing Medical Education: Educating Nonpsychiatric Practitioners About Sexual Misconduct

Medical education is a lifelong process, and the content of instructional approaches to sexual misconduct for physicians who have completed their training is not strikingly different from that proposed for undergraduate and graduate medical education. One mistake frequently made in unsuccessful continuing medical education programs is the assumption by lecturers that the audience is sophisticated about the universal psychological characteristics of the doctor-patient relationship. Although we do not advocate talking down to an audience, it is important to recall the enormous variability among medical schools regarding education about the doctor-patient relationship. Second, even with appropriate instruction as medical students and residents, many physicians remain uncomfortable about feelings that arise in the context of caring for patients. Unfortunately, except for peer-group supervision there are few ongoing mechanisms for practicing physicians to directly address these issues. The reinforcement of earlier learning about sexual misconduct is not nearly as common as continuing medical education in traditional areas such as diagnosis and treatment of illness. Continuing education about sexual misconduct frequently takes place through pamphlets and newsletters published by state medical licensing agencies and through periodic lectures and courses, often presented as parts of larger general educational meetings. Since state medical boards are regulatory agencies, it is not surprising that education about sexual misconduct for practicing physicians includes much greater emphasis on state laws about the legal consequence of such unethical behavior.

Successful educational offerings for practitioners also attempt to integrate the challenges of daily medical practice. Treating patients after office hours without office staff present, sharing too much of the physician's personal life with his or her patients, the danger of socializing with patients, the hazards of house calls, identification of physician impairment, and the treatment of so-called problem patients (i.e., "angry," "hysterical," or "seductive" patients) are a few of the topics frequently addressed in continuing medical education about physician sexual misconduct.

Lawyers who specialize in medical malpractice and risk management and psychiatrists who consult with state medical boards on physician impairment issues are often invited to address practitioners on sexual misconduct and related issues having to do with the prevention of behavior that violates professional boundaries. The importance and mechanics of seeking early professional consultation when difficult treatment situations arise are also emphasized. Courses on improving communication within the doctor-patient relationship also enhance the practitioner's ability to understand their patients in more sophisticated ways. Many physicians acknowledge the helpfulness of presentations on the stresses of practice, the medical marriage, and the physician as parent as they highlight the psychological vulnerabilities likely to arise among physicians. Finally, in some states like New Mexico, education is coupled with medical licensure by requiring all applicants to appear for an interview, at which time the state laws about sexual misconduct are reviewed with each physician by a state medical board member.

Conclusion

Ethical, legal, and clinical concepts and practice must be taught and reviewed throughout all phases of physicianhood. Although there will always be a small minority of physicians with severe character deficits that make them resistant to educational efforts and who must be forced to discontinue the practice of medicine after sexual involvement with patients, the vast majority of students, residents, and physicians, we believe, when appropriately informed about the risks of sexual misconduct and its devastating effects on patients, are able to modify practice styles and appreciate in greater depth the complexity of the doctor-patient relationship. Education for the prevention of sexual misconduct at all levels of medical education serves to define the extent of misconduct, foster a greater comfort in openly discussing universal sexual feelings that arise with the doctor-patient relationship, establish strong guidelines about unacceptable boundary violations, and ultimately enhance public awareness regarding the unacceptability of such physician behavior and appropriate legal recourse when unethical physician behavior victimizes patients.

References

American Medical Association, Council on Ethical and Judicial Affairs: Sexual misconduct in the practice of medicine. JAMA 266:2741–2745, 1991

American Psychiatric Association, Subcommittee on Education of Psychiatrists on Ethical Issues: Ethical Concerns About Sexual Involvement Between Psychiatrists and Patients. Videotaped vignettes for discussion. Washington, DC, American Psychiatric Association, 1986

American Psychiatric Association, Subcommittee on Education of Psychiatrists on Ethical Concerns: Reporting Ethical Concerns About Sexual Involvement With Patients. Videotape. Washington, DC, American Psychiatric Association, 1990

American Psychiatric Association: Fact Sheet—Patient/Therapist Sexual Contact. Washington, DC, American Psychiatric Association, April 1992

American Psychiatric Association: Resource Document: Legal Sanctions for Mental Health Professional–Patient Sex. Washington, DC, American Psychiatric Association, 1993

American Psychiatric Association: Principles of Medical Ethics With Annotations Especially Applicable to Psychiatry. Washington, DC, American Psychiatric Association, 1998

Blackshaw SL, Patterson P: The prevention of sexual exploitation of patients: educational issues. Can J Psychiatry 37:350–357, 1992

Bloom JD, Resnik M, Ulwelling JJ, et al: Psychiatric consultation to a state board of medical examiners. Am J Psychiatry 148:1366–1370, 1991

Bouhoutsos J, Holroyd J, Lerman H, et al: Sexual intimacy between psychotherapists and patients. Professional Psychology: Research and Practice 14:185–196, 1983

Bourgeois J, Kay J, Markert R, et al: Medical student abuse: perceptions and experience. Med Educ 27:363–370, 1993

Carr ML, Robinson GE, Stewart DE, et al: Survey of Canadian psychiatric residents' sexual contact with educators and patients: results of a national survey. Am J Psychiatry 145:690–694, 1988

Coverdale J, Bayer T, Isbell P, Moffic S: Are we teaching residents to be ethical? Academic Psychiatry 16:199–205, 1992

CV NOS DR-5289–88 and DR-37–89, DC Super CT (October 29, 1989)

Epstein RS, Simon RI, Kay GG: Assessing boundary violations in psychotherapy: survey results with the Exploitation Index. Bull Menninger Clin 56:1560–1566, 1992

Feldman-Summers S, Jones G: Psychological impacts on sexual contact between therapists or other health care practitioners and their clients. J Consult Clin Psychol 52:1054–1061, 1984

Fisher N, Fahy T: The eroticized consultation: practical and ethical considerations. Compr Ther 18:2–5, 1992

Freud S: Observations on transference-love (1915), in The Standard Edition of the Complete Psychological Works of Sigmund Freud, Vol 12. Translated and edited by Strachey J. London, Hogarth Press, 1958, pp 157–173

Gabbard GO, Nadelson C: Professional boundaries in the physician-patient relationship. JAMA 273:1445–1449, 1995

Gabbard GO, Wilkinson SM: Management of Countertransference With Borderline Patients. Washington, DC, American Psychiatric Press, 1994

Gartrell N, Herman J, Olarte S, et al: Psychiatrist-patient sexual contact: results of a national survey I: prevalence. Am J Psychiatry 143:1126–1131, 1986

Gartrell N, Herman J, Olarte S, et al: Psychiatric residents' sexual contact with educators and patients: results of a national survey. Am J Psychiatry 145:690–694, 1988

Gartrell N, Milliken N, Goodson WH, et al: Physician-patient sexual contact—prevalence and problems. West J Med 157:139–143, 1992

Glaser RD, Thorpe JS: Unethical intimacy: a survey of sexual contact and advances between psychology educators and female graduate students. Am Psychol 41:43–51, 1986

Granich R, Mermin J: Romantic relationship between physicians and patients. Acad Med 67:586, 1992

Gutheil TG, Gabbard GO: The concept of boundaries in clinical practice: theoretical and risk-management dimensions. Am J Psychiatry 150:188–196, 1993

Herman JL: Trauma and Recovery. New York, Basic Books, 1992

Kay J: Traumatic deidealization and the future of medicine. JAMA 263:572–573, 1990

Kardener SH, Fuller M, Mensh IN: A survey of physicians' attitudes and practice regarding erotic and non-erotic contact with patients. Am J Psychiatry 130:1077–1081, 1973

Kluft RP: Treating the patient who has been sexually exploited by a previous therapist. Psychiatr Clin North Am 12:483–500, 1989

Levitt C, Freedman B, Kaczorowski J, et al: Developing an ethics curriculum for a family practice residency. Acad Med 60:907–914, 1994

Miles SH, Weiss-Lane L, Bickel J, et al: Medical ethics education: coming of age. Acad Med 64:705–714, 1989

Notman MT, Nadelson CC: Psychotherapy with patients who have had sexual relations with a previous therapist. J Psychother Pract Res 3:185–193, 1994

Perkins HS: Teaching medical ethics during residency. Acad Med 64:262–266, 1989

Pope KS: Teacher-student intimacy, in Sexual Exploitation in Professional Relationships. Edited by Gabbard GO. Washington, DC, American Psychiatric Press, 1989

Pope K, Bouhoutsos J: Sexual Intimacy Between Therapists and Patients. New York, Praeger, 1986

Rest JR: Can ethics be taught in professional schools? The psychological research. Ethics: Easier Said Than Done 1:22–26, 1988

Robinson WL, Reid PJ: Sexual intimacies in psychology residents. Professional Psychology: Research and Practice 16:512–520, 1985

Roman B, Kay J: Residency education on the prevention of physician-patient sexual misconduct. Academic Psychiatry 21:26–34, 1997

Self DJ, Baldwin DC, Wolinsky FD: Evaluation of teaching medical ethics by an assessment of moral reasoning. Med Educ 26:178–184, 1992

Self DJ, Schrader DE, Baldwin DC, et al: The moral development of medical students: a pilot study of the possible influence of medical education. Med Educ 27:26–34, 1993

Sheehan KH, Sheehan DV, White K, et al: A pilot study of medical student abuse: student perceptions of mistreatment and misconduct in medical school. JAMA 263:533–537, 1990

Silver HK, Glicken AD: Medical student observations, incidence, sexuality and significance. JAMA 267:527–532, 1990

Simon RI: Clinical Psychiatry and the Law, 2nd Edition. Washington, DC, American Psychiatric Press, 1992

Sulmasy DP, Geller G, Levine DM, et al: Medical house officers' knowledge, attitudes, and confidence regarding medical ethics. Arch Intern Med 150:2509–2513, 1990

Wagner N: Ethical concerns of medical students. Paper presented at the 1972 Western Workshop of the Center for the Study of Sex Education in Medicine, Santa Barbara, CA, 1972

Wilbers D, Veenstra G, van de Wiel HBM, et al: Sexual contact in the doctor-patient relationship in the Netherlands. BMJ 304:1531–1534, 1992

SECTION IV

Therapeutic and Rehabilitative Issues

8

SEXUAL MISCONDUCT AND THE VICTIM/SURVIVOR
A Look From the Inside Out

Janet W. Wohlberg, M.S., A.B.D.,
Deane B. McCraith, M.S., O.T.R./L., L.M.F.T.,
and Dolores R. Thomas, M.S.W., L.I.C.S.W.

Professional literature on sexual misconduct by health care professionals[1] is extensive. With few exceptions, however (e.g., Bantau 1987; Gifford 1987; Linda 1987; Siegel 1986, 1987), the voices of ac-

We thank Nancy Avery, Estelle Disch, Linda Jorgenson, and Linda Weisberg for their helpful input and comments on this manuscript.

[1]"Health care professionals" includes all psychotherapists and counselors, physicians with specialties other than psychotherapy, and clergy who practice counseling. Approximately 85% of participants in the Boston victim/survivor group were abused by psychotherapists; 10%, by clergy; and the remainder, by physicians with other specialties.

knowledged victim/survivors of sexual misconduct and exploitation have been largely missing.[2] In addition, papers accepted by the professional community as highly authoritative on the topic have often depended on victim/survivor populations of fewer than 20 to reach conclusions about the nature of the abuse and the characteristics of victims (e.g., Apfel and Simon 1986; Dahlberg 1970; Smith 1977) and on abuser populations of fewer than five to reach conclusions regarding their characteristics (e.g., Celenza 1991). Whereas many authors have demonstrated impressive insights into the problem, despite the difficulties of studying the phenomenon on a reasonably comprehensive scale, much of the professional literature nonetheless raises both anger and anxiety from victim/survivors who feel unrepresented, misunderstood, and invalidated by authors' apparent needs to tightly categorize victim/survivors using popular professional nomenclature (e.g., Gutheil 1989; Smith 1984). To victim/survivors, such categorization is also often perceived as "blaming the victim."

Adding to the frustration of victim/survivors is the fact that much of the literature is the work of subsequent treaters who, because of the very nature of their role and whatever countertransferential issues are raised by the fact of the abuse—and because a victim/survivor may be denying the extent of the impact of the abuse and/or minimizing or not reporting the abuse—tend not to be able to separate and diagnose the characteristics of a victim/survivor into those that existed before the abusive relationship and those that came about as its result. "Although we had met twice a week for three years," says Deborah T., "I never felt safe enough to raise the issue of the sexual abuse with my previous therapist. It remained a secret, and I was left alone to bear the shame I felt."

The perspective of subsequent treaters is additionally complicated by the frequent tendency of victim/survivors to move from therapist to therapist, often not staying long enough for a subsequent treater to observe the patient healing and returning to a state of emotional equilibrium.

Among the clear exceptions to the above have been writings by re-

---

[2]We are aware of a considerable number of scholarly papers, theses, etc. that have been prepared by authors whose interests in the topic have arisen from direct personal experiences but who have written through the voices of researchers.

searchers at the Walk-In Counseling Center (WICC) in Minneapolis (e.g., Schoener et al. 1989), where by 1989 staff members had provided consultation to more than 1,000 people who presented with the complaint of having been sexually exploited by mental health professionals. WICC is thus looked to by many in the victim/survivor community as a reliable resource, and WICC's findings are generally consistent with our experiences as participants in the extensive Greater Boston victim/survivor network.

Our intent in writing this chapter is to present a personalized perspective based on our own experiences and on our collective contacts with more than 500 victim/survivors and victim/survivor groups from throughout the English-speaking world, including the United States, Canada, England, Australia, and New Zealand.

Victim/Survivor Terminology of Self-Identification

One often emotionally charged debate within the victim/survivor community concerns how to self-identify. Pam S., whose therapist sexually exploited her over a 12-year period, refers to herself as a "survivor." A professional woman, Pam says, "I don't want to go through life thinking of myself as a victim. I don't want that to be my expectation of myself. I want to believe that what happened to me is over and that I have the power to see to it that it doesn't happen again." For Pam, the term *survivor* emphasizes that healing and empowerment are possible. It suggests that, despite the harm that was done to her, she has taken back her life, and she is now in control.

Alice H., sexually exploited by the therapist to whom she turned when her only child was run over and killed by a school bus, prefers the term "victim." "Survivor feels too much like the Holocaust or incest," she says. "I was victimized, and to me there's no shame in that. Everyone gets victimized at one time or another. I've pretty much healed from it, but that doesn't change the fact that I was a victim of Dr. X." For Alice, the term *victim* emphasizes that a violation was committed, that harm was done, that she was an innocent participant who was in the proverbial "wrong place at the wrong time," and that she wishes to make clear that the blame and responsibility lie squarely and unequivocally with the perpetrator.

Because we have not observed any relationship between the term chosen by an individual and the type of abuse, its duration, or factor other than possibly the stage of healing, and because our attempt is to represent a wide range of the community, we have elected to use the composite term *victim/survivor.*

It is important for subsequent treaters to establish, soon after the revelation of abuse, how the patient self-identifies in order to better understand his or her state of mind. At some of the early stages of healing, when victim/survivors are experiencing ambivalence weighted in the direction of loving and protective feelings toward the abuser, or feeling confusion and guilt over responsibility for what took place, it is not unusual for them to use broad and generalized terms that display a lack of clarity concerning their role in the abusive relationship. At these early stages, it is probable that neither term, *victim* or *survivor,* will be a comfortable fit, as the pain from the abuse may feel insoluble. It is also not unusual at these early stages for the victim/survivor to characterize the relationship as "an affair."

It is in this latter terminology—that is, the use of the word *affair*—that we all too often see complicity of subsequent treaters with victim/survivors. *Affair* suggests at least equal responsibility for what has taken place and, worse, may promote the victim/survivor's self-image as evil seducer. It is critical for subsequent treaters to firmly but calmly drive a change in the victim/survivor's nomenclature by making clear from the very earliest points that what took place was not an "affair," that what took place was wrong, and that it was the therapist's responsibility to have seen to it that sexualization of the prior therapy did not occur. Working with the victim/survivor to establish a more comfortable and appropriate term for the relationship should prove useful in helping the victim/survivor gain a healthier perspective of what occurred.

Who Is the Victim/Survivor?

Schoener et al. (1989) have concluded, as have we, that development of a narrow typology of the woman or man who becomes a victim of sexual abuse in a therapeutic situation is not possible (p. 45):

There are no data in the literature to show that any client characteristic predicts sexual involvement with a therapist. Although sexual involvement often has some predictable effects on clients, I do not believe that a clear pattern or syndrome can be found across the board in victims and thus I must reject the notion of a "client-therapist sex syndrome" that was proposed by Pope and Bouhoutsos (1986). Many of the characteristics they noted are also characteristics of other syndromes or victims in general, and we see great variability among victims.

By 1990, Pope appeared to have abandoned the concept of "client-therapist sex syndrome," noting that (p. 485)

Although various clinical (e.g., borderline personality disorder) and historical (e.g., history of incest) factors have been suggested as placing a patient at greater risk for sexual involvement with a therapist . . . , no research published in peer-reviewed journals has provided support for this notion.

A casual survey of more than 400 women in the Boston-based resourcing and referral victim/survivor network TELL (Therapy Exploitation Link Line) affirms Pope's and Schoener's conclusions. These victim/survivors initially entered therapy for every possible reason—death in the family, physical illness, depression, childhood abuse or other trauma, marital problems, etc. Some entered with current situational problems, others with long histories of coping with trauma. For those of us in the TELL network, the only commonality we can find is that we have been in enough pain and sufficiently vulnerable to seek therapy and risk trusting a mental health professional.

There is a virtually endless list of socioeconomic variables as well: some victim/survivors in the TELL network hold advanced degrees, including doctorates in areas such as medicine, education, and psychology, whereas some others have not finished high school. Victim/survivors include those on welfare as well as multimillionaires. We are professionals, entrepreneurs, managers, professors, clerks, writers, manual laborers, nannies, homemakers, and unemployed. We have, among us, participants in all of the major Western religions, as well as atheists and agnostics. We are straight, gay, and bisexual; obese, thin, and average; short, tall, and everything in between. Remarkably few of us wear extreme clothing or hair styles, use large amounts of makeup or perfume, or in any way look or act the role of the "seductress." Chances are you would not notice us on the street, and unless we told you, you would not be aware of the trauma we have experienced.

Although it feels as if there is a disproportionate number of survivors of childhood sexual abuse among us in the victim/survivor network (approximately one-third[3]), the percentages are consistent with the prevalence within the population at large as shown by the outcomes of more than half a dozen surveys taken between 1940 and 1987 (Butler 1985; Haugaard and Repucci 1989; Herman 1981). The findings of these surveys are that between approximately 10% and 60% of adult women experienced some form of childhood sexual abuse, with survey results varying according to the instrument and definitions used and the population studied. Of three large-scale surveys, a 1983 study by Russell, a 1984 Canadian survey, and a 1985 study by Wyatt revealed rates of childhood sexual abuse of females at 38%, 28%, and 59%, respectively.

It stands to reason that the kind of trauma produced by childhood sexual abuse provides a motivation to seek therapy. As noted by Herman (1981, p. 7):

> Female children are regularly subjected to sexual assaults by adult males who are part of their intimate social world. The aggressors are not outcasts and strangers; they are neighbors, family friends, uncles, cousins, stepfathers, and fathers. To be sexually exploited by a known and trusted adult is a central and formative experience in the lives of countless women.

However, even if the percentage of women who experience childhood sexual abuse and who later seek treatment is disproportionate to

---

[3]This is based on observations of self-reports by participants at monthly TELL meetings and through telephone interviews; it has not been studied scientifically. However, our observations are clearly inconsistent with the findings of Smith (1984). Sociologist Estelle Disch, cofounder of the Boston-based group BASTA, estimates that of the close to 500 victim/survivors who have attended her workshops worldwide or who have turned to her for consultation, up to 50% may have experienced childhood sexual abuse. However, Boston social worker and BASTA cofounder Nancy Avery estimates the rate at only 30% of the nearly 120 victim/survivors she has seen in her intensive 12-week workshops, and Attorney Linda Jorgenson of Cambridge, Massachusetts estimates that of her more than 200 victim/survivor clients, the rate of prior childhood sexual abuse is "not more than 30%."

the percentage of the total female population that seeks treatment, and this makes them more likely to be available for exploitation in the therapeutic setting, our estimates still show rates of prior childhood sexual abuse among our victim/survivor population as being no greater than that in the population at large.

Despite this, we still do not know for sure whether prior childhood sexual abuse makes one more likely to experience sexual abuse once in a therapeutic setting, in part because it is possible that such prior trauma makes the victim/survivor of therapist abuse more likely to "keep the secret" and less likely to come forward to our network. Nevertheless, we reject Kluft's (1990) "sitting duck syndrome,"—that is, that previously abused people may be extremely susceptible to subsequent abuse—as too narrow a response to who is going to be abused and why.

What we do know is that anything that blurs boundaries in relationships, whether situational or long-standing, creates an environment in which exploitation is possible and perhaps particularly difficult for the patient to recognize. As Boston social worker Linda K. Weisberg (personal communication, January 26, 1994) wryly observes, "Patients often seek therapy because they have boundary issues; they just don't expect that the therapist will join them."

The area in which we have observed some commonalties is among the several victim/survivors of certain multiple abusers. In 1990, onlookers were startled by the physical resemblance of two victim/survivors of the same therapist who discovered one another at a TELL gathering. In age, height, build, and even hairstyle and voice tone, these women could easily have passed for siblings. When months later a third victim/survivor of the same therapist appeared, this third woman also bore striking physical similarities to the other two. Another perpetrator, Dr. I., specialized in the treatment of women with life-threatening or disfiguring diseases. Of the 17 or more known victim/survivors of Dr. I.'s abuse, all shared this characteristic.

Aspects of the Abuser

If there is no clear profile of the victim/survivor, other than the vulnerability that has brought him or her into the striking range of a potential perpetrator, then what are the likely predictors that a patient will be abused? Although we agree with Bates and Brodsky (1989, p. 141) that "[t]he best single predictor of exploitation in therapy is a therapist who has exploited another patient in the past," it is important to recognize that our current oversight and regulatory systems do not allow us to have ready access to information regarding who has abused, and victim/survivors do not come forward in great enough numbers. It is estimated that only 4%–8% ever report (Strasburger et al. 1992). Even when perpetrators have received significant publicity, the individual and collective memories of the public are short. In states where perpetrators who have lost their licenses are still able to continue to practice, there is little if any protection for the unsuspecting patient who takes at face value the power and legitimacy of the professional's title.

In addition, the transition from potential abuser to abuser is apt to be insidious (Simon 1989), and this potential may only be discoverable through close and careful scrutiny of the potential abuser's personal boundary system, perhaps even before professional training has begun. We recognize that such scrutiny is unlikely to take place.

Individuals who demonstrate highly narcissistic tendencies, appear to be unclear about appropriate relationships with authority figures, display angry or cynical personality traits, or rationalize dishonest and/or unethical behavior may be at high risk to abuse. But these cannot be counted on as indicators, because there are certainly individuals with these traits who are not known to have abused, and many abusers are charming, warm, and highly sociable. More than once we have heard from professionals about their abusing colleagues, "I've known Dr. P. all of my professional career, and I know he would never do such a thing." (For further discussion of the characteristics of abusers, see Gabbard 1989; Gonsiorek 1987; Kottler 1986; Schoener et al. 1989; Simon 1987)

The most prevalent characteristic among perpetrators described to us is their abuse of power and control. Edelwich and Brodsky (1991, p. 40) note that

A major aspect of the clinician's power is symbolized by the fact that it is he or she who reads the client's file, not the client who reads the clinician's file. The saying "knowledge is power" is particularly apt when applied to the privileged information revealed in therapy. This knowledge confers upon the clinician not only an intangible personal advantage in the relationship with the client, but a practical kind of leverage as well. For the therapist not only reads the client's file, but also adds to it, and what is added may have a lot to do with whether the client is discharged from a psychiatric hospital, gets a job, or goes to prison. Power, then, lies in both the possession and communication of confidential information.

In this power lies the potential for abuse.

In cases of overt sexual exploitation of patients involving some form of penetration, the actual sex act appears to be merely a symbol and perhaps the culmination of the abuser's ultimate control of and power over the patient.

Reports of victim/survivors doing secretarial or household chores and/or personal errands for their abusers abound, and it has not been unusual to hear of victim/survivors performing these and other services in the role of slave or servant to master.

When Dr. L. went on vacation with his wife, he would fly Patti M. to the vacation site, put her up in a nearby hotel, and there she would wait to perform oral sex on him one or more times per day. His visits were irregular, and he would become verbally abusive and threatening if Patti was not immediately available upon his arrival.

Susan G. changed from a full-time to a part-time job in order to spend the balance of her time managing her abuser's books, typing his papers, and handling his personal correspondence and bill-paying. All of this was done without remuneration.

Jean T. served dinner and washed dishes for a number of her abuser's dinner parties. This, too, was without pay.

Alan B. was instructed to have sex with a number of his abuser's other patients if therapy was to continue and he was to get well.

Shelly T. was "fined" by her abuser in amounts up to $500 an instance for each time she broke his often ill-defined or unspoken rules. "This is the only way you're going to learn," he told her.

Virginia C. supplied free office space to her abuser in a building she owned, as well as other free services, while paying him for therapy.

Discussion of two additional indicators of power and control as motivator to abuse appear to be largely missing from the literature: In our victim/survivor community, there have been a number of cases of lesbian women coerced into sexual relationships with male therapists, heterosexual women drawn into sexual relationships with lesbian therapists, and similar configurations among male patients. For these victim/survivors, sexual identity is thrown into turmoil and becomes one more aspect of the patient's personality and life that is controlled by the abuser.

Marcia D., married and with a child, left her marriage and moved in with her abuser, who ultimately terminated the 7-year relationship and required Marcia to leave the house they shared. "She told me I was a lesbian and that what was wrong with my life was that I was in denial," Marcia says. "Then she told me to get out of her life. Now I don't know who I am. My husband would like to get back together with me, but I don't know whether I'm straight or gay, and I don't want to hurt him any more than I already have."

There is a high frequency of victim/survivors reporting that their abusers have been sexually dysfunctional, with the sex act taking the form of "servicing" the abuser. In more than half of the incidences that our victim/survivor population reports as having involved penetration, oral sex was the norm.

Jane W.'s abuser, Dr. S., insisted to her that he was unable to participate in vaginal sex due to an inguinal hernia, while another of Dr. S.'s victims reported having had occasional vaginal sex with him despite his stated preference for oral sex. (At his subsequent hearing before the Board of Registration in Medicine, Dr. S. asked for clemency on the basis that his hernia repair had left him impotent, and he was thus no longer a threat to patients. The board was apparently unsympathetic but gave him the option of resigning his license rather than having it revoked.)

Recognition of the Abuser's Power and Ability to Control

Even professionals who understand the power of transference often have trouble believing that such extreme abuses of power can take place without the "consent" of the patient, so it is not surprising that victim/survivors, their families, and their friends generally fail to understand how such abuse can take place, particularly over a prolonged period. For the victim/survivor, this only adds to and confirms the shame, self-blame, and extreme confusion over what has taken place.

At a professional conference at which one victim/survivor related what had happened to her, a psychiatrist in the audience challenged, "You're an obviously intelligent and educated woman. Why would you give your psychiatrist oral sex if you didn't want to?" Other victim/survivors report having been told by relatives, friends, and subsequent treaters, "you should feel flattered"; "I'm sure Dr. X would never do such a thing"; and "it was just his maternal countertransference."

The words of Deborah T., as she describes her reentry into therapy, are especially poignant:

> I had not been in treatment for 7 years subsequent to my being abused by my former therapist. At that time, I felt that what had occurred with my therapist had been my fault; that I had seduced him, and I was a consenting adult. I felt shame and humiliation, that no one would understand or believe me, or that they, too, would view it as my fault . . . . During our first session, I raised issues around my sexual fantasies about her . . . . she responded negatively. She said she could not understand why I would be feeling this way, since I did not even know her . . . . I was left feeling embarrassed and rejected . . . . I continued the therapy but never again raised my sexual feelings and fantasies.

As healing takes place, and the victim/survivor becomes more likely to report and share what has happened with subsequent treaters, family members, and friends, it is critical that the victim/survivor's story be believed and validated. For those of us in the victim/survivor community, the prevalence of incidents of servitude and coercion into unwanted and undesired acts is so great, presented in such graphic detail, and told with such overwhelming shame and embarrassment, that we have little doubt that most, if not all, actually occurred. It is probably for this reason that Boston social worker and Harvard professor Nancy Avery (1993) noted, "There is nothing any therapist can do for a victim/survivor that comes close to what another victim/survivor can do." For a victim/survivor, knowing even one other victim/survivor can validate the experience and break the isolation.

For the vulnerable patient, the concept of "consent" is meaningless. Abusing therapists rely on the vulnerability of a patient and the strength of the transference not only to coerce the sexual relationship but also to avoid its disclosure. Dozens of victim/survivors in our network report having been told, "If you tell anyone, I won't be able to continue to see you"; "You might damage my reputation"; or "We have to be careful that my wife doesn't find out." Some abusers have used their power with even more menacing threats and actions:

Martha W. was told, "If you tell anyone about us, I'll simply say that you were hallucinating."

Peg C.'s abuser used his power to undermine her attempts to be admitted into a graduate school program. Although he willingly agreed to supply a letter of recommendation for her, she later learned that he recommended that the school not take her due to her "emotional instability."

Diane M. says, "I was regularly told by Dr. Z. that if I did anything to jeopardize the relationship, I would look like the one at fault because no one would question the word of a respected doctor over mine. He also told me that I might ruin his reputation. Since I, as a 'sick' patient, needed the sexual therapy he offered, he had to protect himself from any unfortunate false understandings or allegations on my part. He made me promise to keep our relationship a secret, indicating that this protected both of us from public misunderstanding."

Victim/survivors are fearful of the power of their abusers, even well after the abusive relationship has ended, and often refrain from reporting the abuse because of it. Victim/survivors report having dreams in which they are harmed or even killed by their abusers, and while many acknowledge that there is no rational basis for the fear, it remains prominent and paralyzing.

Victim/survivors who themselves are therapists particularly fear being characterized by their fellow therapists as "damaged goods." Because much of the abuse of therapists by therapists takes place under the guise of collegiality and involves a senior clinician with a trainee or neophyte, these victim/survivors believe that they will have little credibility against the word of their abuser and, furthermore, that their abuser will characterize them to the professional community as "crazy" or inept.

"If this gets out," said Regina C., "I'll never get another referral from anyone. He knows everyone, and everyone respects him. He can really ruin me in this community, and I know him, he will." (See also Edelwich and Brodsky 1991; and Luepker and Schoener 1989, for a further discussion of the power dynamics in psychotherapeutic relationships.)

Married victim/survivors often have another worry—that the abuser will tell a spouse and/or children what has taken place. Many spouses interpret the abuse as their own victimization, not just by the therapist—which it is—but by their mate as well. Such spouses blame the victim/survivor for marital infidelity and often experience jealous rage. Questions such as, "Why did you have oral sex with him when you've always refused to have it with me?" are not uncommon. Thus the victim/survivor who fears his or her spouse learning about the abusive relationship often does so with significant reason.

Melanie D., guilty over her relationship with her abuser, divorced her husband without ever telling him what happened. She says she still loves her husband and that her husband loves her and is bewildered over what went wrong in their marriage. She fears that if she takes action regarding the abuse, her abuser will tell her husband of the relationship.

Other victim/survivors have reported being fearful that their children, parents, or friends will be told, and of the possibility that physical harm will be done to themselves and their families. At least a dozen of the victim/survivors in the TELL network reported that their abusers claimed to have ties to organized crime, to have dangerous patients who would do their bidding, or to have connections to professional killers. Two victim/survivors reported having their car tires slashed and believe it to have been done as a warning by their abusers. So great may be the fear of retaliation that it is common for the patient to protect the abuser rather than to risk further victimization.

If there is any single fear that victim/survivors almost universally hold, it is that their abusers—who, despite their abusive behavior, are still seen as holding superior knowledge and power to declare what does or does not constitute mental health—will say that the victim/survivor is "crazy," and that the victim/survivor will be unable to know whether this is true or not. Reassurances from a subsequent treater may do much to mitigate this feeling of lack of trust in oneself, but the fears of being crazy are often so deeply implanted by the abuser that substantial healing must take place before this fear is dissipated. This is all the more reason for a subsequent treater to acknowledge the reality of what has happened and help the victim/survivor recognize that, although the abusive situation was crazy and inappropriate, this does not mean that the victim/survivor is. Often, meeting another victim/survivor of the same abuser will help to bring about a healthier perspective and self-image as the two compare notes and realize that the insanity was within the abuser, not themselves. Therefore, encouraging and supporting the victim/survivor's efforts to locate and communicate with other victim/survivors may be an important element of certain stages of subsequent treatment.

Patterns of Abuse

We have noted three patterns of abuse reported by victim/survivors: serial, cluster, and intermittent. Three women abused by Dr. R. discovered that he had a pattern of perpetrating in a serial fashion, and two of his victim/survivors were able to establish that he had begun to have sex with one within a week of terminating his relationship with the other. Cluster abusers perpetrate abuse on a number of patients at the same time.

Jennifer M. was told by her abuser that when his office shades were drawn, it meant he was having sex with another patient. In addition to the fact that he drew the shades when he was having sex with Jennifer, she became further convinced of the veracity of this statement some time later on meeting another of her abuser's patients. Intermittent abusers appear to abuse a single patient at a time with a substantial period of inactivity in between. However, due to the nature of the therapeutic relationship, which takes place behind closed doors, and the reluctance with which victim/survivors come forward, we cannot fully know what the actual patterns are. It is unclear to us whether there are single-episode abusers, although we accept the possibility. In a number of situations, we have been able to locate victim/survivors of an abuser for whom the time lag between incident reports is 10 years or more.

Degree of Harm

It is increasingly our belief that no one gets through the experience of being sexually abused and exploited by a therapist unscathed, although a number of factors appear to us to determine the degree of harm done. What happened in the sexually exploitative relationship, when it occurred, how often, how it affected other relationships, and its meaning differ greatly among victim/survivors. It is important, therefore, for subsequent treaters to avoid making assumptions, even assumptions based on studies of the existing literature, as to what the needs of a victim/survivor might be. Instead, it is crucial that subsequent treaters be open and willing to listen, believe, and give support, recognizing that each victim/survivor has unique circumstances and needs and that therapy is a dynamic process.

Variables or mitigating factors that may function individually or in combination to determine the degree of harm from the exploitative relationship may include age at the time of abuse, duration of the abusive relationship, emotional stability at presentation and preabusive stages of the therapy, the strength of the victim/survivor's family and/or social network, previous history of abuse, and the degree of marker-event trauma that caused the victim/survivor to seek therapy. The degree of the abuse itself, characterized somewhat crudely by many in the victim/survivor community as "whether or not he put it in," does not seem to add to or lessen the amount of harm. As more than one victim/survivor has noted, "abuse is abuse," and more subtle boundary violations, which may or may not precede actual intercourse, can be devastating for many. Attorneys Linda Jorgenson and Pamela Sutherland (1993) note that although jurors can understand and become angry at therapists who have sexual contact with their patients, it is actually not the sex act that inflicts harm on the patient, but rather the symbolic meaning of the sexual contact as well as other boundary violations that breach trust.

We have found that abuse that does not involve sexualized physical contact (hugging, kissing, petting, stimulation) and/or penetration can actually cause a greater degree of harm, particularly because in its aftermath the victim/survivor's experience is often discounted by subsequent treaters, family, and friends as something that actually never took place. The victim/survivor of noncontact abuse also has little if any recourse through legal or professional channels. The rewards of having gotten out of the abusive relationship before contact took place may be far outweighed by the severe breach of trust that has been experienced and the subsequent invalidation of the feelings aroused.

Age at the time of abuse appears to be one of the most critical factors determining the degree of harm. It is painful to witness the agony of women, now adults, who were sexually exploited by therapists during their early adolescent and teen years. For them, the abuse appears to have been committed with the approval of their parents, who most likely selected the therapist, paid for the therapist's services, and often accompanied the child to the therapy hour, sitting in the waiting room while the child was being abused just yards away.

Helene S. describes just such a scenario in vivid detail. "I never said anything to my parents because I assumed they must have known what was going on. They were right outside the door, even when he put me into the hospital and had sex with me and then gave me shock therapy. I got more and more depressed and found it harder and harder to function, and they just kept taking me back to him."

Mary T., now 48, recalls being hospitalized by her parents for depression at age 16. In 1992, the therapist who had abused her each time he entered her hospital room 32 years earlier finally lost his license. More than two dozen women had come forward to say that he had also abused them. For Mary, her abuse is still a "dirty secret." She has not told her husband, has only recently shared what had happened to her with her subsequent treater, and her one conversation with another victim/survivor of her abuser ended with her refusal to join the others in bringing charges against him.

Often by the time these victim/survivors recognize the damage that has been done to them and have begun to heal enough to take legal action, such as bringing civil litigation or complaints before licensing boards, they are thwarted by statutes of limitation and inability to locate the abuser, who may have died or moved to a different state or country. Other forms of action, such as talking publicly about the abuse, often result in listeners characterizing what took place as "ancient history" and discounting the impact with comments such as "What's the big deal? You're all right now." Inability to confront the abuser leaves the victim with traces of distrust in her sense of reality and lingering questions about what actually took place.

When family and social networks are strong, damage may be mitigated by support, understanding, and a shared anger over what has taken place. When Jane W. told her teenage daughter about the abuse and her intent to take action, her daughter's response was, "Get the bastard." "I was surprised," says Jane. "I thought she'd be embarrassed, but she wasn't. She was just angry that someone had done that to me. I felt validated and cared for." Others among Jane's family and friends had similar reactions, enough so that the few negative comments had little damaging impact on Jane's self-esteem and ability to move forward and take action.

Within the victim/survivor network are those whose abusive relationships lasted up to 25 years, along the way destroying marriages, dividing child from parent, and severely undermining the patient's ability to form relationships with anyone other than the abuser. Extended abuse compounds feelings of complicity, feelings exacerbated by reactions such as "Well, you must have wanted it to let it go on that long" and "You could have gotten out if you had wanted to" when the abuse is revealed to subsequent treaters, family, and friends. Patients in long-term (6 months or longer) abusive relationships become conditioned to believe that the sexual abuse is therapeutic and that the sexual encounters with the therapist will alleviate depression, increase self-esteem, and even help with a troubled marriage. Given the therapist's increasingly powerful role as a father figure, patients doubt themselves rather than question the abuser's support or risk losing the abuser's support as they themselves become ever more dependent.

Effects of the Abuse

Effects of sexual abuse in psychotherapeutic settings vary according to the victim/survivor's history and experience. However, certain effects are virtually universal, and most are well reported in the current literature (e.g., Gartrell et al. 1989; Schoener et al. 1989).

Undermining of Trust

The undermining of trust is perhaps the most pervasive and comprehensive effect. Victim/survivors not only stop trusting those around them, including coworkers, children, spouses, and subsequent treaters, they also stop trusting themselves. Victim/survivors report having problems differentiating between reality and fantasy and also trusting their abilities to make intelligent decisions, particularly about keeping themselves safe. This may lead to avoiding subsequent therapy or a pattern of "therapist shopping." It is not unusual for victim/survivors to go through as many as a dozen therapists, seeing most for fewer than three sessions, before making a commitment. Gina S. saw 17.

Deborah T. describes trusting neither herself nor her subsequent treater: "I have come to understand how unconsciously I was setting the stage to test whether my relationship with Dr. K. would be safe or if I would be able to seduce him like I felt I had done with my previous male therapist. Beginning therapy again was terrifying for me, although I had little awareness of the terror I was feeling. Trusting this new therapist . . . to be therapeutic and not abusive seemed almost impossible."

Diane M. noted, "I had gone through seven different therapists and finally concluded that if I had to trust someone, I would never get anywhere. I decided to give up on trusting anyone and just work on the issues."

Ambivalence

Victim/survivors experience ambivalent feelings about themselves, the abuser, and the abuse. This ambivalence can last long after the abusive relationship has ended, and even beyond the point at which action against the abuser has been undertaken and completed. Although a victim/survivor experiences anger and confusion over what has taken place, it is often difficult for him or her to give up the belief that the abuser cared deeply about him or her, and to let go of the memories of having been wanted by and sexually involved with someone of such power. This is especially true for victim/survivors who have lost virtually all other relationships or who have been thwarted in making relational commitments to others during the relationship and are thus left alone, with no framework within which to measure their self-worth.

Isolation

The isolation of patients by their abusers is systematic and perhaps even calculated to set up the relationship and keep it a secret. In the process, victim/survivors often become alienated from their families and friends, and divorce from an otherwise loved spouse is not infrequent.

Gail G., an artist who had begun to experience some commercial success with a number of one-woman shows at prominent galleries, was told by her abuser to stay away from her boyfriend because he wasn't good enough for her. Next, her abuser told her that her family clearly made her depressed and that she would get sicker if she continued to see them. Friends, coworkers, and virtually everyone in Gail's social network was systematically excised from her life. Finally, her abuser told her, "You're not a very good artist. Why don't you find something you can do well?" "In the end," says Gail, "all that was left was him." Today Gail is a librarian.

Other Effects

In addition to the effects described above, victim/survivors experience extreme guilt and shame over what has taken place; fear; depression that may range from mild to suicidal thoughts and behavior; rage, often undirected and uncontrolled, toward the abuser, self, and others; and symptoms of posttraumatic stress disorder, including inability to concentrate, nightmares, and flashbacks. Most victim/survivors report experiencing at least four effects.

Reports of suicide attempts among those in the victim/survivor community are prevalent, but we will probably never know how widespread this reaction is because of the inability to accurately track those who succeed.

Recovery and the Recovery Process

The good news for the victim/survivor community is that healing from abuse in psychotherapeutic settings is possible. Appropriate subsequent treatment and networking with other victim/survivors are important elements of the recovery process. The therapist who wishes to provide subsequent treatment must recognize that each victim/survivor will have a different set of needs, personal history, and experiences. Thus, the subsequent treater must avoid stereotypes and refrain from imposing expectations. A knowledgeable subsequent treater who understands sexual misconduct and malpractice reporting options and processes should be better able to support a victim/survivor through a healing process, particularly if that healing process is to include taking action.

At the initial contact, the subsequent treater should clarify the patient's agenda, assess the patient's current needs, and also recognize that asking a victim/survivor to trust him or her is probably an impossible request. Even mildly suggesting that trust of the therapist is a critical part of the treatment will likely send the victim/survivor running, not walking out the door, since for most, the constant admonition of the abuser is likely to have been, "you'll just have to trust me." Therefore, the subsequent treater must assume mistrust, validate the experience, and make clear what the boundaries will be in the subsequent treatment. In addition, subsequent treaters should be cognizant of the reservoir of love and caring that the victim/survivor may continue to feel for the abuser and thus be cautious about characterizing the abuser in extreme and negative terms.

During the first phase of treatment, healing from the abuse should serve as the focus. It is important to help victim/survivors understand their options, support the telling of the story and exposing of the secret, and undertake grief work as the victim/survivor begins to work through the anger, ambivalence, and loss. Among the therapy goals of this phase are to help the victim/survivor acknowledge the betrayal, violation, and loss that has been experienced, end the isolation by helping the victim/survivor to network and become connected, dispel guilt and shame, restore trust, channel anger and rage, reclaim personal power and self-esteem, and put the experience into a realistic perspective. For many victim/survivors, this phase of treatment is painfully slow and frustrating, often taking years, and considerable backsliding may be experienced.

Phase two of therapy—that is, dealing with the problems for which the patient originally sought help and examining earlier life themes— may be inextricably intertwined with phase one and may or may not be necessary or part of the client's agenda. It is also possible that until these earlier issues are addressed, resolution of the abuse may not take place, since they are inherently tied together.

Taking action, such as mediation, reporting to a medical board or professional ethics committee, bringing legal charges, or speaking out publicly, may supply an additional and important route to healing for many victim/survivors. When and if a victim/survivor elects to take a particular course of action, it is important for subsequent treaters to understand the process and the implications for the therapy and to help the victim/survivor gain a perspective and understanding of the emotions aroused. Many victim/survivors feel frustrated and disempowered at a number of points in the process, particularly when a lawyer is unwilling or unable to deal with the emotional turmoil of a client or an ethics committee is unresponsive or vague. Attorney Linda Jorgenson (personal communication, January 27, 1994) suggests that taking action is an opportunity for reempowerment and that attorneys representing victim/survivors can play an important role. "Part of making them [the victim/survivors] whole again," she says, "is having them involved in the process if that is what they want to do."

Winning through a legal process, whether through settlement or trial, must be recognized as having potentially complex outcomes. "At trial time," says Jorgenson, "when the jury comes in with the verdict, victim/survivors are usually absolutely elated. Then there is a crash." For the victim/survivor, a tremendous amount of energy has gone into a process that may have taken 3 years or more. The victim/survivor's personal identity and life's cause may have become intensely caught up in the process, and reports of depression and even attempts at suicide are common when the process has been completed. Some victim/survivors elect to extend their activities by doing something to help the field; for example, funding research or conferences, writing, and speaking out. For many, the money awarded through the legal process feels "dirty" and perhaps, at some level, unfulfilling and undeserved. Jorgenson postulates that this reaction "goes back to not having resolved issues around their responsibility for the relationship." With additional work in subsequent therapy, victim/survivors may begin to think about the financial reward as tangible evidence of the validity of the wrong that has been done to them.

Many abusers who elect to take a combative or defensive route fail to understand what victim/survivors generally want. As Lorraine M. says, "An apology would be nice." Says Jorgenson, "Sometimes when they get exactly what they want, for example compensation, apology, and acknowledgment of the wrong that has been done, without a battle, they feel validated, particularly when proof of the abuse would have been difficult. However, when proof is not difficult, abusers' apologies are generally hollow."

Victim/survivors appear to take one of two routes after resolving the issues around sexual abuse in psychotherapeutic settings: Some want to put the experience behind them and move on. Others take up what we have elected to title "the victim/survivor's mission," trying to lend support to others.

Conclusions

We do not believe that sexual abuse of patients by members of the health care professions is going to go away, and we believe that few, if any, perpetrators can be rehabilitated. It is probably part of the human condition that at least some of those in positions of power are going to abuse it. However, we believe that by sensitizing the overwhelming percentage of members of the health care professions who would not perpetrate such abuse, and by educating the consuming public, we can do much to slow the rate as well as to support those who fall victim to such abuse.

References

Apfel R, Simon B: Sexualized therapy: causes and consequences, in Sexual Exploitation of Patients by Health Professionals. Edited by Burgess AW, Hartman CR. New York, Praeger, 1986, pp 143–151

Avery N: The impact of sexual abuse by therapists. Presented at The Consortium Training Program on Boundary Issues and Therapy Abuse, Pittsfield, MA, May 13, 1993

Bantau A: Another victim speaks. California Psychologist 22(4):11, 1987

Bates CM, Brodsky AM: Sex in the Therapy Hour: A Case of Professional Incest. New York, Guilford, 1989

Butler S: Conspiracy of Silence: The Trauma of Incest. Volcano, CA, Volcano Press, 1985

Celenza A: The misuse of countertransference love in sexual intimacies between therapists and patients. Psychoanalytic Psychology 8(4):501–509, 1991

Dahlberg CC: Sexual contact between client and therapist. Contemporary Psychoanalysis, Spring 1970, pp 107–124

Edelwich J, Brodsky A: Sexual Dilemmas for the Helping Professional. New York, Brunner/Mazel, 1991

Gabbard GO: Sexual Exploitation in Professional Relationships. Washington, DC, American Psychiatric Press, 1989

Gartrell N, Herman J, Olarte S, et al: Prevalence of psychiatrist-patient sexual contact, in Sexual Exploitation in Professional Relationships. Edited by Gabbard GO. Washington, DC, American Psychiatric Press, 1989

Gifford L: The victim speaks. California Psychologist 22(4):11–12, 1987

Gonsiorek JC: Intervening with psychotherapists who sexually exploit clients, in Innovations in Clinical Practice. Vol 6. Edited by Keller PA, Heyman SR. Sarasota, FL, Professional Resource Exchange, 1987, pp 417–427

Gutheil TG: Borderline personality disorder, boundary violations, and patient-therapist sex: medicolegal pitfalls. Am J Psychiatry 146(5):597–602, 1989

Haugaard JJ, Repucci ND: The Sexual Abuse of Children. San Francisco, CA, Jossey-Bass, 1989

Herman JL: Father-Daughter Incest. Cambridge, MA, Harvard University Press, 1981

Jorgenson LM, Sutherland P: Psychotherapist liability: what's sex got to do with it? Trial, May 1993, pp 22–25

Kluft RP: Incest and subsequent revictimization: the case of therapist-patient sexual exploitation with a description of the sitting duck syndrome, in Incest-Related Syndromes of Adult Psychopathology. Edited by Kluft R. Washington, DC, American Psychiatric Press, 1990

Kottler J: On Being a Therapist. San Francisco, CA, Jossey-Bass, 1986

Linda J: Therapist sexual exploitation of a patient—the patient's perspective. Register Report 14:13–14, 1987

Luepker ET, Schoener GR: Sexual involvement and the abuse of power in psychotherapeutic relationships, in Psychotherapists' Sexual Involvement With Clients: Intervention and Prevention. Edited by Schoener GR, et al. Minneapolis, MN, Walk-In Counseling Center, 1989

Pope KS: Therapist-patient sexual involvement: a review of the research. Clin Psychol Rev 10:477–490, 1990

Pope KS, Bouhoutsos J: Sexual Intimacy Between Therapists and Patients. New York, Praeger, 1986

Schoener GR, Milgrom JH, Gonsiorek JC, et al: Psychotherapists' Sexual Involvement with Clients: Intervention and Prevention. Minneapolis, MN, Walk-In Counseling Center, 1989

Siegel S: Is registration the answer? Psychotherapy Newsletter 4(1):4–6, 1986

Siegel S: About re-evaluation counseling. American Mental Health Counselors Association News 11(2):9, 1987

Simon RI: Clinical Psychiatry and the Law. Washington, DC, American Psychiatric Press, 1987

Simon RI: Sexual exploitation of patients: how it begins before it happens. Psychiatric Annals 19(2):104–112, 1989

Smith S: The golden fantasy. Int J Psychoanal 58(3):311–324, 1977

Smith S: The sexually abused patient and the abusing therapist: a study in sadomasochistic relationships. Psychoanalytic Psychology 1(2):99–112, 1984

Strasburger LH, Jorgenson L, Sutherland P: The prevention of psychotherapist sexual misconduct: avoiding the slippery slope. Am J Psychother 46(4):544–555, 1992

9

PSYCHODYNAMIC APPROACHES TO PHYSICIAN SEXUAL MISCONDUCT

Glen O. Gabbard, M.D.

Sexual misconduct is not a monolithic entity. In some quarters, however, there has been a tendency to politicize physician-patient sex into a highly reductionistic formula: Physicians who engage in sexual activity with patients are evil men preying on helpless female patients (Gutheil and Gabbard 1992). The solution, then, is to throw the "bad apples" out of the profession (Gabbard 1994a, 1994b). This formulation vastly oversimplifies a multifaceted and complex professional problem, but it has considerable appeal to those who embrace it. By labeling one subgroup as incorrigible and utterly evil, these physicians can reassure themselves that sexual misconduct is behavior that occurs only among "impaired physicians" who have "character disorders" and are therefore completely different from the rest of us.

As one who has been extensively involved in the evaluation and treatment of physicians charged with sexual misconduct, I suggest that such a view is inherently dangerous. By projectively disavowing our own vulnerability to boundary transgressions with patients, we may become complacent and fail to monitor our own feelings toward patients. A more sensible and eminently more practical approach to the problem is to assume that we are all vulnerable to various boundary transgressions and take appropriate measures to prevent acting on strong feelings toward patients.

The Council on Ethical and Judicial Affairs of the American Medical Association (AMA) concluded that "sexual contact or a romantic relationship concurrent with the physician-patient relationship is unethical" (Council on Ethical and Judicial Affairs 1991, p. 2741). Within this broad ethical code, a wide range of actions are considered unethical. On one end of the continuum we find the unscrupulous, predatory physician who anesthetizes women in his office and rapes them while they are unconscious. On the other end of the continuum we would find situations in which a small-town family practitioner is faced with the dilemma that he is the only physician in town and anyone he might wish to date is also his patient. Because he does not want to remain single, he may ask one of his patients out on a date and start a romantic relationship. Although each of these practitioners is acting unethically according to the AMA code, a psychodynamic evaluation would reveal a different diagnostic understanding and a different rehabilitation plan based on the significant differences between them. This diversity among practitioners brings us to a basic principle that applies to the evaluation and treatment planning of all instances of sexual misconduct: the development of an individually tailored treatment and rehabilitation plan follows from a thorough psychiatric assessment of the practitioner in question (Gabbard 1994b; Schoener et al. 1989).

Psychodynamic Classification

In my own clinical experience of evaluating, treating, and consulting on many cases of physician sexual misconduct, I have found that the vast majority of the physicians involved fall into four psychodynamically based categories: 1) lovesickness, 2) masochistic surrender, 3) predatory psychopathy and paraphilias, and 4) psychotic disorders (Gabbard 1994a, 1994b). The reader should keep in mind, however, that within each of these categories there is considerable individual variation based on the unique psychodynamic features of the physician involved. Nonetheless, this classification is useful, not only in terms of understanding the motivations of the physician, but also in planning and implementing rehabilitation efforts.

Lovesickness

Many physicians who are charged with sexual misconduct explain their behavior by saying they are "in love" with the patient. Love, of course, is irrelevant to ethical considerations when considering sexual boundary violations. Nevertheless, in the throes of lovesickness, many physicians believe that standard ethical codes do not apply to them and will argue that it may be unethical for *other* physicians to have sex with their patients but that somehow their case is different.

A typical profile of the lovesick physician involves a middle-aged male physician who has been swept off his feet by a much younger female patient and who himself is in the midst of significant problems in his own marriage or personal relationships (Brodsky 1989; Gabbard 1991, 1994a; Twemlow and Gabbard 1989). However, female physicians who become sexually involved with patients most commonly fit into this category as well. A variety of DSM-IV (American Psychiatric Association 1994) diagnoses may be found in lovesick physicians. Some have mild depressions or are basically healthy but experiencing a severe life crisis. Others suffer from obsessive-compulsive, borderline, or histrionic personality disorders or from less severe forms of narcissistic character pathology.

Masochistic Surrender

Many physicians pride themselves on their tireless and selfless devotion to their patients (Gabbard 1985). These self-sacrificing features leave these physicians vulnerable to manipulation by severely disturbed patients who make unceasing demands for special treatment. In a typical scenario, the physician masochistically submits to the patient's tormenting demands by violating one nonsexual boundary after another, leading to a progressive descent down a "slippery slope" of boundary violations until the relationship is sexualized (Gutheil and Gabbard 1993; Strasburger et al. 1992). DSM-IV diagnoses in this group include obsessive-compulsive personality disorder and dependent personality disorder, and the controversial diagnosis of self-defeating personality disorder, which is not included in DSM-IV.

Physicians are often highly conflicted about the expression of aggression. Indeed, their whole professional demeanor involves a reaction formation against it. They assiduously avoid any appearance of being cruel, sadistic, or hateful by constantly ministering to the needs of others. As a result, they may feel that to set limits on patients' demands is an unacceptable act of aggression. Certain kinds of patients, including incest victims, somatizers, and those with borderline personality disorder or dissociative disorders, may induce guilt in physicians about being unresponsive to their patients' needs. Patients may accuse the physician, for example, of not really caring about them but simply working like a prostitute who only pretends to care because she is receiving a fee.

The poignant demand by such patients to be rescued resonates with powerful rescue fantasies that may reside in the physician's unconscious. These rescue fantasies may lead to a therapeutic zeal that ignores professional boundaries in the service of meeting the patient's needs. The doctor may go to the patient's home in the middle of the night for a "house call," may stop charging a fee, may hold the patient and hug her to comfort her while she cries, and may disclose aspects of his own life with the best of intentions. The patient soon reveals herself as an insatiable and bottomless pit of longings, and the physician discovers that none of his ministrations seem to soothe the patient's despair. She may threaten to kill herself if he does not continue to gratify her every wish. The ultimate wish may be a sexual relationship.

Predatory Psychopathy and Paraphilias

Another group of physicians, overwhelmingly male, account for much of the highly sensationalized media coverage of sexual misconduct. These practitioners view the doctor-patient relationship as an ideal setting in which to gratify their sexual wishes. The behavior may take many forms. The doctor may perform a breast examination on a female patient who presents with a complaint of an earache. The doctor may anesthetize patients in his office and rape them while they are on the examining table. In more extreme situations the physician may inquire about the patient's most horrific sexual fears and then suggest that they act them out together as a way of helping her work through her anxiety.

The medical profession would prefer to believe that such practitioners could not make it through medical school and residency and establish themselves in medical practice. However, a small but worrisome number of physicians do indeed become licensed practitioners despite their serious character pathology. After sexual misconduct comes to light, investigations of these practitioners' backgrounds often reveal histories of various kinds of corruption—cheating on examinations, criminal charges, falsifying medical records, and so forth. In many instances, a faculty member may "blow the whistle" on one of these trainees, only to back down after the young physician threatens to sue the institution if he were to be expelled. In hopes of avoiding a lawsuit, training committees often reluctantly decide that it would be better simply to graduate the trainee and hope that he practices in another state.

Predatory psychopathy, as used here, is a category much broader than DSM-IV antisocial personality disorder. It refers to a specific kind of *behavior* that is psychopathic. Some physicians who manifest this behavior are diagnosable as having severe narcissistic personality disorders with antisocial features. Although all doctors with paraphilias are certainly not antisocial, those who act on their perverse tendencies with patients have significantly compromised superegos as well as character pathology similar to those of psychopathic predators. Physicians in this group frequently have been involved with a number of different patients and, before the advent of the National Practitioner Data Bank, often moved from state to state so they could continue to practice.

Psychotic Disorders

The rarest category of the four is psychosis. Although the excuse of being temporarily psychotic is occasionally used by psychopathic predators to avoid legal consequences, the actual number of physicians who engage in sexual misconduct because of a psychotic process is quite small. One female resident became manic and thought the television set was telling her that she had the power to cure schizophrenia through love. She helped a male schizophrenic patient elope from the hospital where she worked and had sex with him in an effort to cure him. She went on a chaotic cross-country trip in her car and repeatedly had sex with the patient. She was later hospitalized and prescribed lithium.

Psychodynamic Treatment Considerations

Before any form of treatment or rehabilitation can be begun, an individual psychiatric assessment is required in the evaluation of every physician. If the physician adamantly denies the charges, there is no point in proceeding with a treatment or rehabilitation plan because it will be a waste of time, energy, and money for all concerned (Gabbard 1994a; Schoener et al. 1989). If the physician acknowledges the sexual transgression, then a thorough diagnostic assessment should allow a tentative judgment about which of the four categories captures the physician's major psychodynamic features.

Beyond categorization, however, the task of evaluation is to *understand* the physician. Integral to the psychodynamic approach is the notion that each person is unique and complex, and therefore a physician's behavior has distinctive meanings. An individualized treatment/rehabilitation plan is designed to address the unique needs of each physician.

A typical rehabilitation plan may include any or all of the following features (Gabbard 1994b): 1) pharmacotherapy (if indicated), 2) assignment of a rehabilitation coordinator, 3) personal psychotherapy, 4) practice limitations, 5) supervision, and 6) further education and training regarding professional boundaries and professional conduct.

Pharmacotherapy

Pharmacotherapy should not be considered antithetical to a psychodynamic approach. Indeed, medication and psychodynamic psychotherapy often work synergistically and result in improvements that neither modality alone could achieve (Gabbard 1992; Luborsky et al. 1993). Many physicians become depressed and even seriously suicidal after being charged with sexual misconduct. They may require a combined treatment approach that relies on antidepressant medication to address vegetative symptoms (such as psychomotor retardation, loss of appetite, insomnia, and anhedonia) while psychotherapy addresses issues of self-esteem and interpersonal difficulties.

Dr. A was a 67-year-old gastroenterologist who had been accused of sexual misconduct after he hugged a young female patient and kissed her on the forehead. The patient, who had been a victim of childhood sexual abuse, experienced it as an assault. Dr. A explained that he had been taught to be fatherly and caring toward his patients and was shattered by the charges. When he came for evaluation by a psychiatrist who consulted with the licensing board, Dr. A told the psychiatrist, "My life is over." He went on to say that he had closed his office and retired. With his children grown and his practice gone, he saw no reason to keep on living. When the evaluating psychiatrist asked Dr. A if he was thinking about killing himself, his response was, "I don't see any reason not to." He was given fluoxetine 20 mg a day and briefly hospitalized until he seemed less suicidal and somewhat more hopeful about the future. Psychotherapy was also started while he was on the inpatient unit.

Assignment of a Rehabilitation Coordinator

A rehabilitation coordinator is usually a physician assigned by the licensing board or an impaired physicians organization of the state. This individual has overall responsibility for the implementation and coordination of the rehabilitation plan. The physician in this role should be knowledgeable about problems of sexual misconduct and rehabilitation approaches. In general, he or she should not be selected by the physician who is charged with sexual misconduct. There have been instances in which the rehabilitation coordinator is chosen by the physician/patient because of a mutual friendship between the two. They may play golf together or socialize regularly with their spouses. The accused physician feels that his colleague will "go easy" on him and be biased in his favor. Rehabilitation under such circumstances can be a sham.

The rehabilitation coordinator, if a psychiatrist, may take charge of prescribing psychotropic medication for the accused physician. However, in the ideal situation, the rehabilitation coordinator should not be serving in the role of the psychotherapist. A central task of the rehabilitation coordinator is to make regular reports to the licensing board or impaired physicians committee responsible for the rehabilitation program. With the coordinator also serving as the doctor's psychotherapist, confidentiality is seriously compromised, and the patient may feel like he or she cannot open up and speak honestly with the therapist for fear that any information may be passed on to the board.

Dr. B was a 42-year-old male family practitioner who had been charged with doing unnecessary breast examinations by three different female patients. As part of his rehabilitation plan, he saw a psychiatrist once weekly who served as his psychotherapist and also reported to the Board of Healing Arts regarding his progress in rehabilitation. These reports were made quarterly in a lengthy letter that described the psychotherapy process and the patient's behavior at the office. Dr. B had to have a female chaperone present when examining women, so that no unethical behavior would take place during the physical examinations he performed. However, the psychotherapy process was at a stalemate. Dr. B would show up for appointments but would rarely talk about any material relevant to his sexual thoughts, feelings, or behavior. In response to direct questions, Dr. B would acknowledge that he had intercourse with his wife and occasionally masturbated. However, he would provide no further information about sexual fantasies, feelings toward patients, or temptations at the office. When his psychotherapist asked him about his reticence, he repeatedly said, "Everything I say in here can be used against me."

As the case of Dr. B illustrates, psychotherapy can become a meaningless exercise in futility if the doctor/patient has no assurance of confidentiality. One of the key components of a psychotherapeutic contract is that the patient can say whatever he or she wants to without severe consequences. When that contractual understanding is removed because the psychotherapist and the rehabilitation coordinator are the same person, the process takes on a legalistic ambiance, and the therapist may feel more like a law enforcement officer than a clinician (Gabbard 1995).

Some state boards and impaired physicians committees find it too expensive or too cumbersome to split the functions of psychotherapist and coordinator. Others worry that unless the psychotherapist is reporting, sexual misconduct may be recurring and the board would have no way of knowing about it. Some therapists compromise by telling the physician/patient that he or she will break confidentiality and report to the board *only* if sexual boundary violations are repeated. Even this compromise, however, can encourage concealment or dishonesty in the process. The primary task of the psychotherapist must be to understand the patient, and a trusting relationship cannot be based on a "double-agent" status of the psychotherapist.

This perception of double-agentry in the therapist is simply an exaggerated form of a transference issue that is pervasive in the psychotherapy of physicians charged with sexual misconduct (Gabbard 1995). Patients always suspect that the therapist may *really* be working for the board rather than for them. In cases where reporting to the board is required, the issue is less one of transference distortion and more of an accurate perception of the situation.

The psychotherapist may also feel like an extension of the board who is charged with policing the profession. This corresponding countertransference experience is heightened when the psychotherapist feels a primary obligation to the licensing board or his profession rather than to the patient. Most therapists must constantly monitor this aspect of countertransference, because if it is allowed to develop unchecked, the therapist may unwittingly convey moral condemnation toward the patient. This attitude will interfere with the patient's freedom to share disturbing thoughts, feelings, and impulses.

Psychiatrists can make a contribution to ending this controversy by educating licensing boards about the necessity of confidentiality to make such psychotherapy viable. A reasonable position for the licensing board to take is to ensure that quality treatment is provided to the physician being rehabilitated. The board does not need to know the content of that treatment if they know that the psychotherapist is competent in psychodynamic therapy and in the implementation of rehabilitation plans in general.

Personal Psychotherapy

In the psychodynamic approach to rehabilitation, psychodynamic psychotherapy is obviously the linchpin around which the rest of the plan revolves. Nevertheless, a key aspect of a psychodynamically based evaluation is the determination of suitability for psychotherapeutic work. If the accused physician has no remorse, no motivation to change, and no recognition that his behavior is wrong, then psychotherapy is contraindicated. Licensing boards have notorious problems in rehabilitating physicians who have features of the psychopathic predator, and these frustrations have contributed to the increasing trend in many states toward criminalization of doctor-patient sexual relations. Many experts in the field have concluded that because certain physicians are refractory to rehabilitative efforts, the safest approach is to lock them up so they can do no harm to future patients.

Some predatory physicians readily catch on to what the evaluating psychiatrist is looking for and may present a convincing performance that persuades the examiner that the accused physician is suitable for psychotherapy. When such physicians enter into a psychotherapeutic relationship, they may be able to "go through the motions" without making any fundamental change, as described in the following vignette:

Dr. C was a 38-year-old male gynecologist who had been charged by several patients with a variety of behaviors falling under the category of sexual misconduct. He would frequently perform a pelvic examination in such a manner that his thumb stimulated the patient's clitoris. He would then make comments to the patient such as, "You seem to be enjoying this too much. This is supposed to be an exam." He also asked several patients if they would like to join him for a drink after work. Several women also complained that after completing the pelvic examination, he stood between their legs for a long time as he talked to them, to the point where they felt violated by his behavior. Still others complained that he would rub their backs seductively while talking to them about their history and complaints.

When Dr. C started psychotherapy, he told his therapist that he was interested in understanding why this pattern came up again and again with women because his goal was to be faithful to his wife and not attempt to gratify his needs with patients. He spoke at length about his childhood and how his mother had been seductive with him. Whenever the therapist made an observation or offered a bit of insight, Dr. C would make comments such as, "I never thought of that before," or "That's a very helpful thought."

Things appeared to be progressing well until his therapist heard from the licensing board that Dr. C had been charged with another episode of sexual misconduct that had occurred only a week before. Dr. C's therapist confronted him with his failure to mention the episode in therapy. Dr. C erupted in a rage at his therapist and screamed, "It's none of your goddamn business! You and the licensing board have no right to tell me who I can or cannot date. All these women want me—I don't force anything on them. I don't need treatment! This is pure bullshit!"

This brief vignette illustrates the need of the psychotherapist to periodically reassess whether the patient is truly suitable or is simply complying with expectations and "working the system." In this case, Dr. C was reevaluated by the board and had his license suspended.

Physicians who fall into the other categories may or may not benefit from psychotherapy. Motivation to understand and change their behavior is obviously a key predictor of positive response to such treatment. Some lovesick physicians may initially be unsuitable for psychotherapy because they do not believe that anything unethical occurred. They feel that their love for their patient has transcended any ethical considerations and wonder why "falling in love" requires treatment. However, when the infatuation wears off, they are often remorseful, reflective, and highly motivated for psychotherapy. Many of the lovesick physicians and most of the masochistic surrender types have good potential for rehabilitation.

Approximately half of the physicians charged with sexual misconduct are not amenable to rehabilitation, in my experience, because of severe character pathology, lack of motivation to change, and dishonesty. Some physicians with paraphilias who may be unsuitable for dynamic psychotherapy may be responsive to 12-step approaches that use an addiction model, but even in those settings, only about half the physicians appear to have the potential for rehabilitation (R. Irons, personal communication, August 1994).

Effective psychodynamic therapy with physicians who have been charged with sexual misconduct must begin with careful attention to the therapeutic alliance. The psychotherapist must create an atmosphere of nonjudgmental acceptance so that the patient can express his or her misgivings about punishment and rehabilitation. Most physicians come to psychotherapy after having received certain disciplinary sanctions that they may feel are not fair. Even though rehabilitation is intended to be separate from disciplinary actions, the patient may begin with the feeling that it is an extension of the punishment meted out by the board for his behavior. Clarification of the reality of the situation may help as well as straightforward education about the psychotherapist's role. An important element of forging an alliance is to be certain that the therapist and the patient are collaborating around consensually held goals for the treatment. A frequent problem is that the therapist's agenda is to focus on the reasons for the sexual misconduct, while other issues may be more prominent in the mind of the physician/ patient. Often a compromise can be reached that encompasses the goals of both parties.

The fundamental goal of psychodynamic psychotherapy in these situations is to uncover unconscious conflicts, relationship patterns, longings, and unmet needs that were determinants in the sexual boundary violations. These issues will emerge naturally in the process if the therapist creates a climate of interested concern and periodically integrates the material from the patient's dreams, associations, transference fantasies, and outside relationships to provide new understanding and insight. A clinical example will illustrate the process.

Dr. D was a 46-year-old family practitioner who worked somewhere between 80 and 90 hours a week and who was recovering from a failed marriage. His wife had recently divorced him because she felt he paid no attention to her needs and had started an extramarital affair with another physician who was a colleague of Dr. D. Reeling from his divorce, he became infatuated with a 27-year-old single female patient who was seeing him for a variety of somatic complaints that did not appear to have a basis in physical disease.

The relationship evolved from an attempt to diagnose and treat her complaints into an effort to rescue her from her misery and finally into a classic lovesick situation in which Dr. D was completely preoccupied with her. He had her move into his apartment with him, and they became lovers. After about 4 months of living together, she broke up with Dr. D and reported him to the State Board of Healing Arts.

After a psychiatric evaluation, he was deemed suitable for rehabilitative efforts and was referred to dynamic psychotherapy. He showed a strong motivation to understand what had happened so that he could master his psychological conflicts and never again transgress boundaries. The therapist asked him how he understood what had happened, and he provided a narrative of how the relationship had evolved. He said that the patient's status as a victim had some form of special appeal to him. She had a history of incestuous sexual relations with her father, and she had been recently dumped by her boss who had had an extramarital affair with her for approximately 18 months. Dr. D had a powerful impression that if she could just find the right man, everything would be fine with her. He recognized that her gastrointestinal complaints and her headaches were probably psychogenic in origin. He noticed that he scheduled her for frequent appointments and spent a longer time with her than he did with other patients.

He poignantly recounted how in one appointment she had told him the details of her incestuous involvement with her father and began to sob. She asked if he would hold her, and he complied. She told him he was the most understanding man she had ever met, and she wished she could find a man like him for herself. She told him how her mother was cold and aloof and how she had had to turn to her father to obtain any sense of being special or loved.

Sensing that the patient's presentation and history must have touched a nerve within Dr. D, the therapist asked him if he felt some kind of special kinship with her. He replied that he too had had a cold and remote mother and had never felt sufficiently loved as a child. He also felt victimized by his wife, who he felt had unfairly dumped him even though he was a good husband. As he continued to talk, Dr. D began to experience a great deal of anger that he had tried to avoid throughout the divorce proceedings. He said he had devoted himself altruistically to serving others, and after all the years of tireless self-sacrifice, his reward was that no one loved him, not even his wife.

The therapist suggested to him that his choice of medicine as a profession might have related to a wish to receive the love and approval from others that he did not receive as a child from his parents. He confirmed that his self-esteem was terribly fragile and that he was extremely needy of affirmation and validation from his patients. He said he was particularly distressed by ungrateful patients who did not seem to appreciate the efforts he went to on their behalf. He said he had a need to be needed, and his patient needed him in a way that he found highly gratifying.

As the therapy continued, the therapist commented that his wish to rescue his patient may have been in some ways a wish to rescue himself because of his strong overidentification with that particular patient. Although he initially questioned that observation, during the next session, he told his therapist that he had thought about it at some length and decided that he was giving to the patient what he himself would like to receive from others. He repeatedly said that his main interest in the patient was not sexual. She provided a sense of validation and affirmation of his goodness that his wife had never provided.

A common theme in the childhood experiences of physicians is the perception that their parents did not provide sufficient love and nurturance (Gabbard and Menninger 1988, 1989). They develop a fantasy that the road to finally winning the parental love and affirmation they long for is relentless self-sacrifice and achievement. Emotional dependency and intimacy may be frightening because they are associated with the fear that one's longings will not be reciprocated. They therefore defend against intimacy and dependency by being *apparently* independent and self-reliant. This reaction formation allows the physicians to see *others* as dependent on *them* instead of acknowledging any dependency in themselves. In the case of Dr. D, his lovesickness was couched in terms of the patient's needing and depending on him as a way of defending against his recognition that he desperately needed the patient's love.

> In his psychotherapy, Dr. D repeatedly expressed conflicted feelings about needing his therapist, and at one point he offered to prescribe some medication for some symptoms of allergic rhinitis that his therapist manifested during the hour. The therapist suggested to him that that would be another form of boundary violation, but he also observed that it might make him feel better if he were giving to his therapist rather than simply taking help from him. Dr. D acknowledged that he was much more comfortable in the role of caregiver.

Elements of the masochistic surrender category were also present in Dr. D. As the therapist uncovered details of the relationship, it became clear that Dr. D had allowed his patient to completely dominate his life. Before they began living together, she would frequently call him at night, and he would go over to her apartment to make "house calls." He did not charge her a fee because she was financially disadvantaged.

The result of approximately 16 months of psychotherapy was that Dr. D could own his dependency needs to a greater degree and integrate them into his life. He found an appropriate woman with whom to pursue a romantic relationship, and he achieved a greater balance between his personal life and his work habits. The case of Dr. D illustrates how important a fulfilling emotional relationship is to prevent the tendency for physicians to satisfy their emotional and sexual needs with patients.

Psychotherapists of physicians charged with sexual misconduct face formidable challenges. Those who choose to treat such physicians are likely to struggle with a sense of outrage by what the physician did to his or her patient. They may also be inclined to feel a countertransference sense of superiority as a way of distancing themselves from the repugnant act. This repugnance may be a defensive posture against an unconscious feeling that "there but for the grace of God go I" (Gabbard 1995). The sexually transgressing physician can easily become a container for the therapist's projectively disavowed, unacceptable impulses.

Another countertransference problem that frequently presents itself is an urge on the part of the psychotherapist to collude with the patient's wish to deny the professional boundaries in the therapist relationship and treat the patient as a colleague. Physicians who have engaged in sexual misconduct may assume that their psychotherapist has the same attitude toward boundaries that they have. They may, for example, casually and informally address their therapist by first name. They may expect "professional courtesy" regarding the fee. They may try to persuade the therapist to develop a social relationship with them and even invite them to play golf or tennis.

This transference wish for special treatment by the therapist deserves careful exploration, because it often reveals major psychodynamic themes. For example, the wish to be treated as special by the therapist may reflect a wish for a special relationship like the one enacted with the patient. The patient's idealization and love may have approximated the longed-for approval that the sexually transgressing physician never received from his parents as a child, as was the case with Dr. D.

Practice Limitations and Supervision

Although the main focus of this chapter is on the principles of psychodynamic psychotherapy in the treatment of sexually transgressing physicians, other structural changes in the practice of the physician may be essential components of rehabilitation. Practice limitations are usually implemented as part of the plan. A psychodynamic evaluation may lead to the conclusion that certain kinds of patients should not be seen by a particular practitioner. For example, Dr. D came to recognize that he had an "Achilles heel" for somatizing sexual abuse victims and avoided them in his practice. Another commonly used practice limitation is a restriction from seeing female patients (if the accused practitioner is male), or the presence of a chaperone in the examining room.

In practice, the stipulation that a chaperone must be present during physical examinations may be more complicated than it sounds. For example, in a solo practitioner's office, a female chaperone is likely to be an employee of the physician. The expectation that she should report any deviation from standard practice is largely unrealistic if she is dependent on the physician's good graces for continued employment. Any reporting of her employer to the licensing board could conceivably result in her losing her job or in her having a strained relationship with the person writing her paycheck.

Supervision on site is often part of the rehabilitation plan and is closely related to practice limitations. In a group practice, the board may stipulate that the physician must have supervision of his or her clinical case load by a designated senior colleague. This process may involve going over every difficult case with the supervisor to be sure that professional boundaries are maintained in the doctor-patient relationship. As noted in the discussion about selection of a rehabilitation coordinator or psychotherapist, the supervisor generally should be chosen by the board rather than allowing the physician to select a close personal friend that he or she believes will be lenient and supportive.

Education and Training Regarding Professional Boundaries and Professional Conduct

Few physicians receive much training in medical school or postgraduate education on the concept of professional boundaries. In a certain percentage of physicians charged with sexual misconduct, the problem is largely one of education. By assigning articles for these physicians to read or suggesting continuing medical education seminars on the subject, they may develop a conceptual framework that helps them determine what is ethical and what is unethical in terms of the doctor-patient relationship.

Concluding Comments

The elements of the rehabilitation plan outlined in this chapter may be supplemented by other measures as needed. The psychiatrist who evaluates the physician may determine that a highly conflicted marriage is an integral part of the sexual misconduct problem and suggest marital therapy as another component of the rehabilitation and treatment plan. This therapy may lead to compromises and concessions that allow the physician to derive greater emotional and sexual gratification from the marriage so that patients are not viewed as potential sources of that gratification. On the other hand, a marital process may lead to a divorce, which may be a positive outcome if the physician is no longer "trapped" in a dead marriage that provides no support. This frees the physician to find more fulfilling relationships with appropriate partners.

Group psychotherapy may also be a highly useful adjunct in some rehabilitation plans. Many impaired physician organizations encourage regular attendance at a meeting of a group of peers so there is a sense of cohesion and collective sharing that helps the physician feel less humiliated and ashamed of the behavior. An impaired physician group generally confers the feeling of acceptance on physicians.

If substance abuse is a complicating factor in the clinical picture, 12-step programs like Alcoholics Anonymous or Narcotics Anonymous may be useful. Many states have specific programs for physicians with substance abuse problems. However, physicians who have committed sexual misconduct but do not have substance abuse problems generally do not do well in such groups because they feel out of place. In some states they are nevertheless assigned to such groups because there are not sufficient numbers of sexual misconduct cases in the physician's geographic area.

A frequent question posed to psychiatrists who are involved in consulting with licensing boards is the optimal duration of the rehabilitation program. How long should the psychotherapy continue? How long should a rehabilitation coordinator be involved? The answer is simple in one sense—as long as the physician needs it. Specific goals for the termination of psychotherapy can be derived collaboratively between the psychotherapist and the patient. The rehabilitation coordinator may wish to be involved well beyond the termination of psychotherapy to be sure that the gains achieved in psychotherapy are consolidated and internalized. The coordinator may only need to meet with the physician quarterly to assess the progress, but a typical duration for the coordinator's involvement is 3–5 years. Some states also request outside consultation from experts in the field to assess the patient's progress and to help determine if rehabilitation is still necessary.

References

American Psychiatric Association: Diagnostic and Statistical Manual of Mental Disorders, 4th Edition. Washington, DC, American Psychiatric Association, 1994

Brodsky AM: Sex between patient and therapist: psychology's data and response, in Sexual Exploitation in Professional Relationships. Edited by Gabbard GO. Washington, DC, American Psychiatric Press, 1989, pp 15–25

Council on Ethical and Judicial Affairs, American Medical Association: Sexual misconduct in the practice of medicine. JAMA 266:2741–2745, 1991

Gabbard GO: The role of compulsiveness in the normal physician. JAMA 254:2926–2929, 1985

Gabbard GO: Psychodynamics of sexual boundary violations. Psychiatric Annals 21:651–655, 1991

Gabbard GO: Psychodynamic psychiatry in the "decade of the brain." Am J Psychiatry 149:991–998, 1992

Gabbard GO: Psychotherapists who transgress sexual boundaries with patients. Bull Menninger Clin 58:124–135, 1994a

Gabbard GO: Sexual misconduct, in American Psychiatric Press Review of Psychiatry, Vol 13. Edited by Oldham JH, Reba MB. Washington, DC, American Psychiatric Press, 1994b, pp 433–456

Gabbard GO: Transference and countertransference in the psychotherapy of therapists charged with sexual misconduct. J Psychother Pract Res 4:10–17, 1995

Gabbard GO, Menninger RW (eds): Medical Marriages. Washington, DC, American Psychiatric Press, 1988

Gabbard GO, Menninger RW: The psychology of postponement in the medical marriage. JAMA 261:2378–2381, 1989

Gutheil TG, Gabbard GO: Obstacles to the dynamic understanding of therapist-patient sexual relations. Am J Psychother 46:515–525, 1992

Gutheil TG, Gabbard GO: The concept of boundaries in clinical practice: theoretical and risk management dimensions. Am J Psychiatry 150:188–196, 1993

Luborsky L, Diguer L, Luborsky E, et al: The efficacy of dynamic psychotherapies: is it true that "everyone has won and all must have prizes"? in Psychodynamic Treatment Research: A Handbook for Clinical Practice, edited by Miller NE, Luborsky L, Barber JP, et al. New York, Basic Books, 1993, pp 497–512

Schoener GR, Milgrom JH, Gonsiorek JC, et al: Psychotherapists' Sexual Involvement With Clients: Intervention and Prevention. Minneapolis, MN, Walk-In Counseling Center, 1989

Strasburger LH, Jorgenson L, Sutherland P: The prevention of psychotherapist sexual misconduct: avoiding the slippery slope. Am J Psychother 46: 544–555, 1992

Twemlow SW, Gabbard GO: The lovesick therapist, in Sexual Exploitation in Professional Relationships. Edited by Gabbard GO. Washington, DC, American Psychiatric Press, 1989, pp 71–87

10

COGNITIVE-BEHAVIORAL TREATMENT OF SEXUAL MISCONDUCT

Gene G. Abel, M.D., and Candice A. Osborn, M.A.

S exual misconduct occurs when a physician crosses a boundary to engage in sexual activities against professional rules of conduct. In general, physicians, violating the Hippocratic Oath, initiate sexual behavior with adult patients.

How do we protect patients?

For more than 20 years, therapists and researchers have been formulating and perfecting treatments that stop perpetrators from committing a variety of sexually inappropriate acts against victims. During this time we have amassed a large body of literature on treating paraphilic behavior. Sexual misconduct fits easily into these treatment modalities because the behavior shares so many similarities with paraphilic behavior.

What may appear confusing is the situational nature of sexual misconduct. Most physicians' sexual misconduct involves behavior that, if initiated with a consenting nonpatient in the privacy of their homes, would be considered acceptable and lawful (i.e., kissing, hugging, touching, intercourse, etc.). This is similar to several situational paraphilias. Frottage (touching of nonconsenting victims), voyeurism (watching nonconsenting victims for sexual gratification), and exhibitionism (exposing one's genitals to nonconsenting victims) are activities that would be quite acceptable if carried out with a consenting partner in the privacy of one's home. In contrast, sexual misconduct —similar to drugging a victim, committing rape, and having sex with a child—involves an unequal power base and the inability of the partner to give consent.

For two individuals to voluntarily consent to sexual interaction, they both must equally be capable of withholding consent without fear of repercussions, must be aware of the possible consequences of the interaction, and must appreciate societal or professional norms for the interaction. This cannot occur when there is an unequal power base between the two individuals, such as adult-child, employer-employee, minister-parishioner, teacher-student, doctor-patient relationships, etc. Patients rarely know the rules established by medical boards for physician conduct with patients; they are also often unaware of the undue influence of their transference toward their physician, or of the negative emotional consequences they will suffer from a sexual relationship with their physician. Within professional relationships there is also the expectation (requirement) that professionals will look out for their patients' best interests, not their own.

Sexual misconduct shares additional similarities with paraphilic behavior. Perpetrators of sexual misconduct and perpetrators of paraphilic acts can commit one episode of inappropriate sexual behavior, but in our experience, once initiated, these individuals continue to engage in the inappropriate behavior. Perpetrators of sexual misconduct, like paraphiliacs, almost universally develop cognitive distortions to rationalize or justify their misconduct. Some perpetrators of sexual misconduct, similar to paraphiliacs, commit misconduct in an attempt to deal with stress, anxiety, depression, substance abuse, or deficits in assertive, social, or sexual skills. Both groups' inappropriate sexual behavior may emanate from personality disorders. In approximately 20% of the sexual misconduct cases in our treatment program, physicians suffer from an actual paraphilia that extends into their medical practice, resulting in sexual misconduct.

Therapists accustomed to providing individual psychotherapy to general psychiatric patients may be uncomfortable with providing therapy to physicians involved in sexual misconduct. In typical individual treatment of the general psychiatric patient, patients anxiously seek resolution to their symptomatology. Physicians who have engaged in sexual misconduct often have no desire to change their behavior, but are seeking therapy at the insistence of their medical board. Most are effective at concealing, having kept their actions secret from their medical colleagues and their families. Their rationalizations and justifications are frequently so extensive that it makes it difficult for the therapist to form the therapeutic alliance so necessary to help change their behavior.

Most sexual misconduct involves male physicians and female patients. Although other forms of misconduct do occur, they are rare. In this chapter, for the sake of brevity, pronouns are used that reflect the most common situation. The reader should understand that there are female physicians who commit sexual misconduct.

The following is a description of an integrated cognitive-behavioral treatment of sexual misconduct (see Table 10–1). It is based on the authors' treatment program for professionals exhibiting a variety of inappropriate sexual behaviors. Unique to this program is the development of extensive checks and balances to ensure adequate supervision of the offending physician and protection of his patients.

Components of Treatment

Identification of the Chain of Antecedent Activities, Stresses, and Emotions Leading to Sexual Misconduct

Physicians involved in sexual misconduct frequently fail to recognize the antecedents to their behavior. Instead, they see their actions as impulsive, unplanned, and unpremeditated—something that just happens. As long as the professional maintains this view he will not be able to organize his life to prevent relapses of the behavior. The physician's denial and avoidance of examining the chain of events help him maintain the myth that his act was impulsive.

Table 10–1.   Sexual misconduct treatment components

A. Cognitive-behavioral therapy

    1. Identification and disruption of the chain of antecedents leading to sexual misconduct

    2. Identification and correction of cognitive distortions supporting sexual misconduct

    3. Building victim empathy

    4. Behavior therapy techniques to decrease paraphilic interests

B. Treatment to resolve emotional conflicts contributing to sexual misconduct

    1. Psychotherapy to treat chronic anxiety, depression, anger, stress, or personality disorders

    2. Skills training to correct assertive and social skills deficits

    3. Bibliotherapy—the physician is required to write a referenced paper on the relationship of his or her emotional problems to sexual misconduct

C. Methods to ensure patient protection

    1. Practice style alterations

        a. Possible restriction of patients served

        b. Physical layout changes to allow monitoring

    2. Specific patient education and protection

        a. Patient's Bill of Rights

        b. Patient survey form

    3. Staff and colleague surveillance systems

        a. Staff and colleague surveillance forms

        b. Sexual misconduct group

        c. Polygraphs

D. Advancement of the physician's practice plan to the licensing board

---

Dr. J. was an overworked midcareer internist engaged in sexual misconduct that included inappropriate examinations, masturbation of female patients, and, on a number of occasions, intercourse with patients. He prided himself on his excessive devotion to his patients, his long hours of work, and the fact that he could complete more technical procedures per day than any of his fellow internists. Although he viewed his actions as impulsive, in actuality, his misconduct followed a rather consistent pattern.

These acts occurred on days when he was exhausted and felt that his long hours justified a reward. Although it was his practice to have a chaperone by his side during procedures, once he had identified the female patient he planned to inappropriately examine, he structured the chaperone's activities so that she was busy with paperwork during the anticipated examination. During these unchaperoned physicals, he spent excessive time talking to the potential victim about her personal life in order to convey caring and concern for her. During the abdominal examination, he would slow down the physical and suggest that he had found something that was not right. He would then tell the patient that a pelvic examination was in order to rule out lower abdominal disease and would position the patient on her hands and knees on the examining table. Conveying his continued concern he would again prolong his bimanual examination. As he became more aroused during the procedure, he would ask the patient to rock back and forth to allow him to better examine her lower abdomen and vaginal area. While she did this, he fantasized about having intercourse with her, imagining the rocking motion as signs of her sexual pleasure.

On completing the examination, he would go to the bathroom, masturbate to thoughts of intercourse with her, return after she had dressed, and spend an excessive amount of time talking with her about his concerns about her health and the results of the pelvic examination, etc. He believed that if he spent extra time with her, the patient was less likely to believe that a portion of the examination was for his own sexual purposes. Between acts of misconduct, Dr. J. avoided thinking about the precursors to his misconduct, since such thoughts would provoke considerable guilt and shame about his behavior.

The therapist can help physicians involved in sexual misconduct learn how to block and obstruct their inappropriate behavior by teaching them to recognize the sequence or chain of events that precede it. Rather than accepting the physician's initial reports that his acts are the result of impulse, the therapist asks for details regarding the setting in which the acts occur; the sequence of events that typically occur; the emotions, feelings, and fantasies that might precede or be concomitant with misconduct; and the post-act emotions, thoughts, and rationalizations. In this case, reducing the physician's work load decreased his exhaustion and the need for "pay-back" from a patient. Demanding that chaperones always be present, irrespective of their other responsibilities, eliminated the privacy necessary to carry out such inappropriate examinations. In addition, the physician was trained in alternative methods of handling dysphoria or emotional upset to resolve this antecedent to his misconduct.

A number of behavioral methods have been developed to help individuals disrupt the chain of events leading to inappropriate sexual behavior. Covert sensitization, ammonia aversion, and imaginal desensitization procedures teach the physician specific steps to take to block these sequences by anticipating negative consequences. Once the strategies are used in vitro, they are practiced in vivo. These specific treatments are described in detail in the literature (Abel and Rouleau 1990; Abel et al. 1984, 1992; Laws and Osborn 1983; Laws et al. 1978; McConaghy 1990; McConaghy et al. 1985).

Cognitive Distortions Supporting Sexual Misconduct

When individuals carry out behaviors inconsistent with their image of themselves, they frequently lose self-esteem and become anxious and depressed. The physician will attempt to neutralize such negative feelings by developing cognitive distortions, justifications, and rationalizations to legitimize his misconduct. Such rationalizations are seen in a variety of criminal acts, in sexually deviant acts, and in over 90% of sexual misconduct cases (Abel et al. 1989, 1992; Smith and Wolfe 1988).

> Dr. A. was a psychiatrist in midcareer who had been having affairs with his patients for over 5 years. He viewed himself as superior to other psychiatrists, whom he saw as distant and remote from their patients. He truly believed that if he showed extreme concern and was sexually intimate with his patients, he could break through their isolation and cure them. He felt immediate empathy for female patients with lengthy histories of suffering excessively because of various interpersonal conflicts or problematic marriages. Boundary violations began as he got physically close to patients during times when they were particularly emotionally upset in his office. He would put his arm around their shoulders, to comfort them. This nonsexual touching eventually extended over time to fondling and, in some cases, sex acts with the patients.
>
> Dr. A. developed a variety of cognitive distortions to justify his be-

havior. Sitting close to patients was not seen as a boundary violation, but as the act of a more caring physician who threw aside traditional rules of therapy conduct to convey greater concern for his patients than other physicians would show. When his patient failed to remove his arm from around her while she was in emotional turmoil, he labeled her behavior as condoning and supporting physical touching as an important aspect of comforting her. When a patient failed to immediately reject his acts of sexual fondling, he interpreted her behavior as accepting his sexual touching as a desired activity between them during the therapeutic alliance. When time had passed without complaints or criminal charges being brought against him, he interpreted the lack of reporting as evidence that his sexual relationships with patients had been so rewarding to the patients that they considered it acceptable. The possibility that his victims had failed to report him because of their shame or their guilt over their participation, or because they had inadequate knowledge about a physician's acceptable behavior never crossed his mind.

Since his actions were secret, he developed his own special thoughts to rationalize away his behavior and never revealed these thoughts to anyone or checked their validity by comparing them to what others might think. Because each physician's faulty cognitions about his inappropriate behavior are so different from those of every other physician involved in sexual misconduct, the stage is set for effective confrontation.

Two methods appear to be especially helpful for disrupting the cognitive distortions of physicians involved in sexual misconduct. First, in a group setting, members are able to confront and correct the irrationality of each other's idiosyncratic faulty beliefs. Thus, when perpetrators discuss the special and unique cognitions they use to rationalize and justify their sexual misconduct, other perpetrators immediately see through the false reasoning.

A second means of confronting and exposing faulty cognitions is to have the perpetrator write a letter (never to be mailed) to one of his victims, explaining in detail all of the ways the physician groomed the patient to eventually involve herself in sexual misconduct. The first draft of such a letter frequently includes apologies from the perpetrator and requests for forgiveness. The perpetrator is asked to remove these elements from the second draft of the letter and to expand on the details of his grooming activity with the individual patient. In addition, this second draft is critiqued to remove all aspects of the victim's behavior that the physician may see as contributing to his misconduct. The final product exclusively focuses on how the physician set up the circumstances that would bring about his sexual misconduct. The process of documenting the way he groomed a patient is highly effective in forcing the physician to break through his rationalizations, justifications, and denial that he violated physician-patient boundaries. Periodically, the physician reviews the final letter. In this way, he attends to the thought processes that he carried out to orchestrate his sexual misconduct.

Readers are referred to writings by Abel et al. (1985), Lange (1986), and Murphy (1990) for further details on the development of cognitive distortions and the role they play in the implementation and maintenance of sexual misconduct.

Deficits in Victim Empathy

Physicians involved in sexual misconduct usually show minimal appreciation of the plight of their victims. This lack of empathy is in sharp contrast to most physicians' perception of themselves as being empathic and concerned about all of their patients. This lack of empathy evolves as the perpetrating physician gradually develops a variety of cognitive distortions to rationalize and justify his behavior. For example, the patient's helplessness and vulnerability motivate the physician to provide help and assistance to the patient. The positive feedback to the physician from the patient who is helped, however, is misconstrued by the physician as being not simply appreciation but a personal message of adoration of the physician, unrelated to the physician's assisting the patient. As the physician interacts with the patient he is allowed to freely ask a variety of intimate questions and, if performing a physical examination, also to examine the patient's body. Physicians involved in sexual misconduct rationalize to themselves that by allowing such questioning and physical examination, the patient is not only allowing the physician the latitude required for medical care but is also demonstrating that she wants and desires this very personal contact with the physician. As the physician explores the patient's sexual history, the patient may believe that she is simply responding to the physician's questions, while the physician himself may perceive that his particular patient wants close, intimate conversation about sexual issues with this particular physician. What transpires is that the physician makes many internal statements to himself justifying and rationalizing his behavior to be consistent with what he hopes or wishes to happen—the patient desiring personal, intimate contact with him. A victim's prior history of sexual abuse, including being victimized by other health care providers, can also impair her ability to confront the physician with his misconduct (Eyman and Gabbard 1991; Feldman-Summers and Jones 1984; Pope 1988).

Perpetrators who are unencumbered by the patient's emotional vulnerability convince themselves that if the patient were upset by his advances, she would simply say so. In actuality, the marked power difference between the physician and the patient, the vulnerability of a patient in emotional turmoil, and the confusion about what constitutes appropriate physician-patient relationships can block the victim's response to misconduct. Unaware that the physician may have been sexually involved with other patients, some victims view the physician's early advances as a loving, caring message and a desire to sustain a relationship.

When misconduct continues, the patient may begin to appreciate that she is being used, and her vulnerability may lessen as she begins to verbalize her dissatisfaction. The physician is usually startled by the feedback he receives and becomes concerned that a malpractice suit may ensue and becomes even more insensitive to the patient.

Treating this lack of victim empathy is further hindered by the reality that exposure of the physician's misconduct frequently brings him into therapy in an adversarial role. Initially, he may focus on cataloging evidence that he has done no wrong to the victim and/or that the victim was an active participant in the sexual encounter. Asking the physician to focus on the consequences for the victim of his actions occurs at the very time the physician is attempting to avoid such issues.

It is startling to see that professionals whose careers allegedly involve helping those in crisis fail to appreciate the feelings, vulnerabilities, and emotional consequences of sexual victimization. This lack of empathy is reinforced because victims may not come to grips with their own anger, hostility, and feelings of being victimized until weeks, months, or even years after the victimization. In most cases, by that time the physician-patient relationship has ceased, so the physician has no opportunity to see the consequences of his behavior. Some patients terminate the relationship in the midst of the physician's grooming them for misconduct, again resulting in the physician failing to get feedback regarding the inappropriateness of such behavior.

A final factor contributing to physicians' lack of empathy for the consequences of sexual abuse is that male physicians, in general, have not been sexual victims. Their own experiences therefore fail to provide them with an adequate appreciation of the emotional consequences of victimization.

To break through the physician's lack of appreciation for the consequences of his behavior for the victim, the perpetrator is asked to read written vignettes or view videotaped vignettes by victims of sexual misconduct and to write summaries of the vignettes with special focus on the patient's feelings, emotions, and interpretation of the events. The physician is then asked to write a summary of an episode of his own misconduct. Victim empathy is further enhanced by having him write a description of this episode from the victim's point of view—that is, from the point of view of the subservient individual in the power relationship. Once again he must focus on appreciating how the victim views the encounter, its emotional impact, and its negative consequences. The physician's therapy continues until he can appropriately empathize with the victim's position.

Paraphilic Interest Leading to Sexual Misconduct

Some sexual misconduct emanates from paraphilic interests. Paraphilic arousal (sexual deviation) may lead to sexual misconduct in the form of frotteurism (in which the perpetrator has an extensive history of arousal to touching or rubbing against women without their permission), exhibitionism, fetishism, pedophilia, voyeurism, sadomasochism, etc. In these cases, the physician typically reports having a lengthy history of specific paraphilic interest and behavior that eventually extends into his medical practice. The majority of cases of sexual misconduct result from nonparaphilic interest, but when paraphilic arousal may be involved, specific steps need to be taken to evaluate the physician for paraphilic interest and, if any is found, to treat it.

Paraphilic interests are generally exaggerations of normal arousal. For example, exhibitionism is a common aspect of normal sexual behavior. An individual shows his body to his partner and seeks a partner who is responsive to him. Exhibitionism, as a paraphilia, is an exaggeration of this characteristic and leads some physicians to expose themselves in an indirect fashion (generally within the context of an error of dressing on the physician's part) so as to experience the same response from a patient that the exhibitionist typically experiences from an unknown victim. All varieties of paraphilias may be expressed in sexual misconduct.

> Dr. C. was early in his career as a psychiatrist. From an early age, he had been specifically attracted to women's breasts, but far in excess of what would be considered normal. His preoccupation with women's breasts constituted a fetishism, although a better term for this would be partialism, when a specific body part becomes overwhelmingly arousing. In medical school, he found himself in a role that allowed him to examine women's breasts as part of the physical examination. He lingered over each breast examination and masturbated afterwards to fantasies of touching and fondling his patients' breasts. Throughout his psychiatric residency, he continued to carry out breast examinations. He would tell patients that antidepressants could cause cardiovascular complications, and then would insist that a physical examination of the chest was essential. During this examination he asked the patient to remove her brassiere and he would touch her breasts.
>
> Once out of his residency, Dr. C. continued breast examinations of his patients. He generally selected a woman of lower socioeconomic status, anticipating that she would be less likely to report him for these inappropriate examinations and believing that, if she did report him, he rather than his victim would be more likely to be believed. When he was reported, he successfully averted charges at three separate practice sites. His supervisors appeared to have been more than happy to drop their pursuit of the allegations as long as he was willing to move to another city to practice.

Paraphilic interest can be directly measured using psychophysiologic assessment. This methodology quantifies the patient's erection responses while the patient views slides of, or listens to audiotaped descriptions of, paraphilic stimuli. The relative power of the paraphilic stimuli is then compared with nonparaphilic stimuli to identify the specific arousal that needs to be treated (Laws and Osborn 1983; Murphy and Barbaree 1988).

Paraphilic interest frequently occurs and is maintained because paraphilic stimuli have become associated and paired with orgasm from an early age. A few events involving actual paraphilic behavior may have served as fantasy material for hundreds or thousands of pairings of paraphilic fantasy with the pleasure of masturbation and orgasm (Abel and Blanchard 1974).

When deviant urges occur, the paraphilic experiences significant anxiety and believes that the only way to relieve this anxiety is to carry out his deviant behavior. One treatment involves teaching the perpetrator relaxation techniques and then having him imagine the anxiety-ridden antecedents to his deviant behavior. By practicing the relaxation methods, he learns to decrease his anxiety through appropriate means. This procedure is repeated until the perpetrator is able to successfully imagine not acting on his urges without concomitant anxiety (McConaghy 1990; McConaghy et al. 1988).

Other forms of cognitive-behavioral therapy have been developed to eradicate the arousal pattern of paraphilic stimuli by having the perpetrator bore himself with the very stimuli that were formerly highly erotic (Abel et al. 1984), by teaching the perpetrator how to pair and associate the paraphilic interest with highly aversive scenes (Abel et al. 1984), or by using an offensive odor (Abel and Rouleau 1990; Maletzky 1980; Maletzky and George 1973).

Unless the role the paraphilia plays in sexual misconduct is appreciated, therapists are likely to assume that the perpetrator's problem is merely poor self-control. Clinical experience, however, indicates that specific therapy targeted at eliminating paraphilic interests is essential to reducing the highly erotically charged stimuli that can prompt some physicians to commit sexual misconduct.

Emotional Conflicts Contributing to Sexual Misconduct

A variety of emotional problems and skills deficits may also contribute to sexual misconduct. Some physicians report reducing their ongoing anxiety and depression by carrying out sexual misconduct. Although such conduct does not resolve basic anxiety, depression, or stress, many physicians see the misconduct as a "quick fix," an immediate method of reducing excessive feelings. Some physicians become involved with their patients because they lack the assertive or social skills necessary to develop satisfying relationships with appropriate adult partners and instead take advantage of the patient's transference to initiate sexual relationships with them. In this way, they relate to patients as if the transference-countertransference between the patient and themselves were real "love," unrelated to the professional relationship. Still other physicians have extensive alcohol and/or drug problems that impair their judgment, allowing them to blur boundaries and engage in unprofessional contact with patients.

Finally, specific personality disorders and intrapsychic conflicts may lead to boundary violations. Narcissistic, dependent, histrionic, antisocial, and borderline personality characteristics are generally lifelong. Examination of the history of these physicians will reveal personality characteristics and related conflicts clearly preceding the sexual misconduct. Misconduct seems to be yet another area in which physicians' personality traits interfere with their functioning.

Psychotherapy.   Treatment for personality disorders that lead to sexual misconduct is no different than that for any patient; this is also true for treatment of chronic anxiety, depression, anger, or stress. Problems of assertive and social skills deficits appear to be especially responsive to classic assertive and social skills training. However, when individual psychotherapy is implemented, this therapist should not also function as the practice monitor (see below). Because of transference and countertransference issues, the therapist providing individual treatment might find it difficult to objectively monitor the physician's practice (Pope 1989).

Bibliotherapy.   Particularly helpful for physicians whose emotional conflicts contribute to their sexual misconduct is the practice of having them complete a literature review that they use to develop a referenced article on the specific area that has been problematic for them. This gives them the opportunity to explore what is already in the literature regarding the specific stressors or conflicts that contribute to their sexual misconduct. For example, a physician whose hypomanic behavior has been a major contributor to sexual misconduct is asked to do a literature search on this topic and to write an article demonstrating his understanding of the interrelationship between hypomania and sexual misconduct. Individuals with narcissistic personalities, drug misuse problems, high denial, or specific paraphilic interests similarly develop referenced articles specific to the antecedent issues leading to their sexual misconduct. When completed, these are then circulated in the sexual misconduct group (see below) and are critiqued, and two or three subsequent drafts evolve until the article reflects the physician's intellectual understanding of the problem.

Practice Changes to Ensure Patient Protection

A major deficiency of programs for treatment of sexual misconduct is the lack of specific steps that protect patients from the physician's potential relapse. When the physician is allowed to return to practice, there is frequently no system set in place that provides close surveillance and supervision of the physician to protect his patients.

Practice style alterations. A number of changes in the physician's practice style will help to reduce the likelihood of relapse. Some physicians' personality characteristics, impulsivity, or boundary limitations are so poor with patients of a specific sex that their practice must exclude those patients. Although physicians with misconduct initially shudder at the possibility of limiting their practice to one gender, by following such limitation they usually report a sense of relief that they no longer have to worry about their sexual urges toward these patients.

Physical layout changes in the office can be particularly helpful to enhance direct monitoring of the physician's interaction with patients. Some surgeons, for example, have altered their physical examination rooms so that all rooms are immediately observable by the nurse. Some physicians have put windows in their office doors or had interconnecting rooms arranged so that a staff member can see the physician at all times, although the patient is precluded from view. Some physicians are restricted to seeing patients only with a chaperone who has been fully informed of the nature of the physician's sexual misconduct and who signs every examination note indicating their presence during the entire examination. In some cases, the physician is permitted to perform patient examinations only in specific rooms and during specific office hours and to conduct hospital rounds only when accompanied by a chaperone.

Alterations in practice style cannot replace cognitive-behavioral treatment for sexual misconduct. Practice style alterations are meant to be an adjunct to therapy to help prevent relapse and to ensure the safety of patients being treated by physicians who have committed sexual misconduct.

Specific patient education and protection. Therapies for physicians involved in sexual misconduct are of course not perfect. Therefore, steps must be included in the physician's total treatment program to protect future patients. Providing future patients with a statement that the physician they have chosen has engaged in sexual misconduct would be an adequate warning for the patient, but such revelations would also drive patients from his practice so that he could no longer function as a physician. Two steps can be taken to educate and gain feedback directly from patients.

First, all patients are provided with a "Patient's Bill of Rights," outlining appropriate and inappropriate conduct between physicians and patients. The Patient's Bill of Rights includes a specific statement that sexual activities between physicians and patients are forbidden during and after treatment, according to the guidelines of the American Psychiatric Association (1998).

A second step involves a patient survey form. The perpetrator and his therapist work out a form similar to the example in Figure 10–1. This form is given out and collected once every 3 months by the physician's office staff and is then sent to the physician's practice plan supervisor. Since uneasiness about the physician-patient relationship, unprofessional behavior, and not feeling at ease with the physician reflect the usual experiences of patients who have been abused, these items are included with more general questions patients are asked to answer regarding their satisfaction with the doctor's practice. Any potential problem areas are investigated by the practice supervisor either with the physician's staff or by the physician's staff interviewing the patients. In this way, checks and balances are put in place to protect the patient/consumer of the physician's practice.

Staff and colleague surveillance system. Too often, when offending physicians are allowed to return to practice, there is no system of surveillance of the physician's practice. When surveillance is required, it is

This questionnaire is designed to give us feedback so we may improve the quality of care rendered to our patients. Your opinions about the treatment you received will help us improve our practice. Please fill in the blanks or circle the response which best describes your opinion.

Today's Date: _____

Your Age: _____

Your Gender: ☐ Male   ☐ Female

Your Name (Optional): _____

Please rate Dr. _____'s performance in the following areas:

		Never	Seldom	Usually	Always
1.	Making me feel comfortable.	1	2	3	4
2.	Explaining the nature and treatment of my surgical problem.	1	2	3	4
3.	Conducting physical examinations professionally.	1	2	3	4
4.	Listening to and understanding my medical symptoms.	1	2	3	4
5.	Having a chaperone present during physical exams.	1	2	3	4

Please rate the office staff in each of the following areas:

6.	Explaining the "Patient's Bill of Rights."	1	2	3	4
7.	Explaining billing procedures.	1	2	3	4
8.	Helpfulness/courtesy.	1	2	3	4

9. What could we do to improve our service to you and/or make you more comfortable?

_____
_____
_____
_____

Please return this form to the Office Manager

Figure 10–1. Patient survey form.

frequently a casual process that does not include specific steps to ensure systematic monitoring of the physician's behavior. Three physician surveillance systems have been developed to correct this deficit.

Staff and colleague surveillance forms similar to the example in Figure 10–2 have been used to check on the physician's functioning. This form is developed by the therapist and the physician to identify the specific inappropriate behaviors the physician has carried out and what actions would have been tipoffs in the past that the physician was grooming a patient for sexual misconduct. Three staff members and/or colleagues are then included in the staff and colleague surveillance system. Participants might include two physicians who provide backup to the perpetrator and one office staff member who interacts continuously with him. These individuals complete forms, similar to those in Figure 10–2, on a monthly basis and advance them to the surveillance monitor. The three individuals who complete monthly reports are not asked to go out of their way to observe the physician. Such "detectives" would soon tire of such a role. Instead, these three observers are asked to learn from the physician the factors that allowed him to carry out sexual misconduct and thereby be more aware of the behaviors that, in the past, have suggested or been correlated with sexual misconduct. To conduct surveillance on a friend or colleague is indeed a difficult task; however, the physicians who have been involved in sexual misconduct have been consistently appreciative and supportive of their surveillance teams. When evidence of possible misconduct is reported on these monthly forms, the therapist contacts the surveillance team member to get greater detail, confronts the physician with his inappropriate behavior in order to correct it, and possibly interviews the physician and his staff.

A second source of physician surveillance is a sexual misconduct group made up of other physicians who have been involved in sexual misconduct. This group is especially helpful because it provides an opportunity for the physician to talk openly with other perpetrators, who are usually in different stages of treatment. These groups can provide useful feedback regarding potential boundary violations, cognitive distortions, and necessary practice changes. Members attend these groups weekly, biweekly, or as infrequently as once every 3 months, depending on where the physicians are in the course of treatment and the extent of misconduct that has occurred.

Rater's Name:_____Date:_____

Rater's Signature: _____

Dr. _____ has been treated for inappropri-
ate sexual touching of adult female patients during examinations. This
behavior might have been recognized because he saw patients without
chaperones, behind locked doors, in settings outside his regular office and
outside regular office hours.

This form is to be completed by his staff or colleagues. Your responses
will be furnished to his medical licensure board, and his therapist.

Please respond to each question accurately.

		Never	Seldom	Usually	Always
1.	The doctor does unnecessary physical exams.	1	2	3	4
2.	Doors are kept unlocked during examinations of all female patients.	1	2	3	4
3.	Female patients are only seen during regular office hours.	1	2	3	4
4.	Female chaperones accompany female patients during exams.	1	2	3	4
5.	The doctor interacts professionally with nurses and staff.	1	2	3	4
6.	The doctor welcomes feedback about his conduct with patients.	1	2	3	4
7.	The doctor maintains professional boundaries with patients.	1	2	3	4

Please add any comments on the back of this page. Dr. _____'s
signature below indicates his awareness and approval of your surveillance
of him and he agrees to your advancing these reports irrespective of their
consequences to him.

_____Physician's Signature

_____Date

Figure 10–2.   Staff and colleague surveillance form.

A final component of surveillance involves the use of polygraphs (Abrams 1989). A major difficulty in evaluating sexual misconduct is that the behavior frequently involves what would constitute normal adult-adult sexual interaction if it occurred outside of the physician-patient context. Traditional psychophysiologic assessment cannot be used to determine whether the perpetrator has engaged in misconduct after participation in therapy. Polygraphy is used to monitor the physician's practice, just as drug screens are used to monitor physicians with drug abuse problems. Once the physician has completed the individual components of treatment and has entered the maintenance portion of treatment, polygraphs are used to identify possible relapses of sexual misconduct. Questions, asked at 6-month intervals, involve any sexual misconduct that has transpired since the patient entered the maintenance phase of therapy or since the last polygraph was obtained.

The use of staff and colleagues and polygraph surveillance might appear to be harsh and excessively intrusive. However, when the physician has already broken traditional boundaries and ethical standards, the trust once enjoyed by that physician is lost forever. Physicians permitted to return to practice have been willing to accept such surveillance, since it allows them the opportunity to continue to practice medicine under conditions that can assure the licensing board that patients are protected.

Advancement of the Physician's Practice Plan to the Licensing Board

Licensing boards have the difficult task of ensuring patient safety while at the same time ensuring that physicians who have committed sexual misconduct are treated fairly. The simplest solution to carrying out such duties is to eliminate the licenses of all physicians involved in sexual misconduct. There are two problems with this approach: first, there is no other profession that demands perfection from their practitioners; second, effective treatment does exist for sexual misconduct. Although a few physicians involved in sexual misconduct have such a plethora of problems that their problems cannot be effectively treated or their practices adequately supervised, most physicians can return to practice with reasonable certainty of safety to their patients. However, state medical boards need assistance in determining how to individualize ad-

equate treatment-surveillance plans. When the total practice plan is
completed, it is advanced to the physician's licensing board for feedback and for a final decision regarding the appropriateness of the practice plan.

Disposition of Cases

No controlled outcome studies on the effectiveness of treatment programs for sexual misconduct exist, and it is unlikely that such studies
will ever be possible, since a control group (physicians involved in sexual misconduct who receive no treatment) is ethically unsound.

The closest we can currently come to outcome studies is to examine
the relapse rates of physicians who have returned to practice once they
have completed treatment. This turns out to be a relatively effective
means of evaluating treatment, since such patients are known to their
medical boards or physician recovery network systems. In the case of
physicians involved in sexual misconduct treated at the Behavioral
Medicine Institute of Atlanta, we have established an extensive feedback system for treatment progress that incorporates a number of individuals who provide information about possible relapse by the
physicians. Furthermore, we frequently use periodic polygraphs to
check the validity of the physician's self-reports that they have been involved in no subsequent misconduct.

Of the cases referred to our treatment program, 52% of the physicians have returned to practice. In fact, the physicians whose cases are
outlined in this chapter have all returned to practice. Of the 48% of
physicians who have not returned to practice, nearly two-thirds of
them were removed from practice either by their medical board or as a
result of criminal action initiated before their entry into our treatment
program. Of the physicians removed from practice before beginning
our treatment program, the majority had become involved with patients outside their office practice (making supervision exceedingly difficult), had impaired decision making as a result of organic disease, or
had criminal charges and/or convictions that precluded their subsequently holding a medical license. Our experience indicates that the
number of patients victimized, the sex of the victims, and the extent
of sexual involvement (voyeuristic activity, fondling, oral or anal sex,
intercourse, or extensive affairs) are not factors determining the accept-

ability of a physician returning to practice. Instead, assuming compliance with treatment, it is primarily the ability to establish a practice plan that protects the public that determines the viability of the physician returning to practice.

At present, physicians completing our sexual misconduct treatment program have a recidivism rate less than 1%. This recidivism rate is markedly lower than that of other inappropriate sexual behaviors, such as the treatment of paraphiliacs. This high success rate probably results from the marked compliance with treatment intervention by physicians; joint efforts by members of the treatment program, the physician's recovery network system, and medical licensing boards; and the fact that most physicians returning to practice have been involved in professional sexual misconduct closely associated with their office practice, thereby allowing close monitoring and supervision once they have returned to practice.

References

Abel GG, Blanchard EB: The role of fantasy in the treatment of sexual deviation. Arch Gen Psychiatry 30(6):467–475, 1974

Abel GG, Rouleau J-L: Male sex offenders, in Handbook of Outpatient Treatment of Adults. Edited by Thase ME, Edelstein BA, Hersen M. New York, Plenum Press, 1990, pp 271–290

Abel GG, Becker JV, Cunningham-Rathner J, et al: The Treatment of Child Molesters. Atlanta, GA, Behavioral Medicine Institute of Atlanta, 1984

Abel GG, Mittelman MS, Becker JV: Sex offenders: results of assessment and recommendations for treatment, in Clinical Criminology: The Assessment and Treatment of Criminal Behavior. Edited by Hersen MH, Hucker SJ, Webster CD. Toronto, M & M Graphics, 1985, pp 191–205

Abel GG, Gore DK, Holland CL, et al: The measurement of the cognitive distortions of child molesters. Annals of Sex Research 2:135–153, 1989

Abel GG, Osborn CA, Anthony D, Gardos P: Current treatments of paraphiliacs. Annual Review of Sex Research 3:255–290, 1992

Abrams S: The Complete Polygraph Handbook. Lexington, MA, Lexington Books, 1989

American Psychiatric Association: Principles of Medical Ethics With Annotations Especially Applicable to Psychiatry. Washington, DC, American Psychiatric Association, 1998

Eyman JR, Gabbard GO: Will therapist-patient sex prevent suicide? Psychiatric Annals 21(11):669–674, 1991

Feldman-Summers S, Jones G: Psychological impact of sexual contact between therapists or other health care practitioners and their clients. J Consult Clin Psychol 52(6):1054–1061, 1984

Lange A: Rational-Emotive Therapy: A Treatment Manual. Tampa, FL, Florida Mental Health Institute, 1986

Laws DR, Osborn CA: How to build and operate a behavioral laboratory to evaluate and treat sexual deviance, in The Sexual Aggressor: Current Perspectives on Treatment. Edited by Greer JG, Stuart IR. New York, Van Nostrand Reinhold, 1983, pp 293–335

Laws DR, Meyer J, Holmen ML: Reduction of sadistic sexual arousal by olfactory aversion: a case study. Behav Res Ther 16:281–285, 1978

Maletzky BM: Self-referred versus court-referred sexually deviant patients: success with assisted covert sensitization. Behavior Therapy 11:306–314, 1980

Maletzky BM, George FS: The treatment of homosexuality by "assisted" covert sensitization. Behav Res Ther 11:655–657, 1973

McConaghy N: Assessment and treatment of sex offenders: the Prince of Wales programme. Aust N Z J Psychiatry 24:175–181, 1990

McConaghy N, Armstrong MS, Blaszczynski A: Expectancy, covert sensitization and imaginal desensitization in compulsive sexuality. Acta Psychiatr Scand 72:176–187, 1985

McConaghy N, Blaszczynski A, Kidson W: Treatment of sex offenders with imaginal desensitization and/or medroxyprogesterone acetate. Acta Psychiatr Scand 77:199–206, 1988

Murphy WD: Assessment and modification of cognitive distortions in sex offenders, in Handbook of Sexual Assault: Issues, Theories and Treatment of the Offender. Edited by Marshall WL, Laws DR, Barbaree HE. New York, Plenum, 1990, pp 331–342

Murphy W, Barbaree HE: Assessment of Sexual Offenders by Measures of Erectile Response: Psychometric Properties and Decision Making. Washington, DC, National Institute of Mental Health, 1988

Pope KS: How clients are harmed by sexual contact with mental health professionals: the syndrome and its prevalence. Journal of Counseling and Development 67:222–226, 1988

Pope KS: Rehabilitation of therapists who have been sexually intimate with a patient, in Sexual Exploitation in Professional Relationships. Edited by Gabbard GO. Washington, DC, American Psychiatric Press, 1989, pp 129–138

Smith TA, Wolfe RW: A treatment model for sexual aggression. Journal of Social Work and Human Sexuality 2:149–164, 1988

11

PSYCHOTHERAPY WITH PATIENTS WHO HAVE HAD SEXUAL RELATIONS WITH A PREVIOUS THERAPIST

Malkah T. Notman, M.D., and
Carol C. Nadelson, M.D.

Many therapists encounter patients who have had a sexual relationship with a previous therapist. Despite knowledge of these liaisons in the professional community, there has been reluctance to acknowledge that these relationships occur and that they are damaging to patients. In this chapter we consider boundary violations, describe the characteristics of therapists and patients in this context, and discuss the clinical aspects of the subsequent treatment of those who

This chapter is adapted from Notman MT, Nadelson CC: "Psychotherapy With Patients Who Have Had Previous Sexual Relations With a Therapist." *The Journal of Psychotherapy Practice and Research* 3:185–193, 1994. Used with permission.

have been sexually abused by therapists, including the transference-countertransference issues that emerge.

The problem of sexual involvement between patient and therapist is receiving greater public and professional attention (Apfel and Simon 1985a; Gabbard and Gabbard 1989; Simon 1991). As awareness of this problem grows, patients are more willing to report these offenses, and there has been increasing pressure on and within professional organizations to intervene and discipline offenders.

In this chapter we consider clinical aspects of boundary violations and the subsequent treatment of patients who have been sexually abused by therapists and other doctors. Although male patient–female therapist and homosexual involvements do occur, the vast majority of cases reported involve a female patient and a male therapist or doctor. Our observations are derived from consultation and treatment of such patients as well as from the experience of one of us (MTN), who participated in a 2-year collaborative effort by members of the Boston Psychoanalytic Society with members of a self-help network of these women.

Clinical Aspects of Boundary Violations

Who Are the Therapists?

There is no one profile of therapists who become sexually involved with patients (Olarte 1991; Pope and Bouhoutsos 1986; Twemlow and Gabbard 1989).

Sometimes therapists who are not exploitative or sociopathic, because of misguided but genuine wishes to be helpful, enter into a sexual relationship that they persuade themselves is in the best interests of the patient. They may respond to a patient's loneliness or feelings of deprivation, believing that they can ameliorate these feelings by gratifying the patient's wishes for "more" of a relationship with the therapist. They may have fantasies about their ability to rescue or transform a patient and may see these gratifications as therapeutic. These beliefs can then progress to sexual relationships, sometimes with the idea, on the part of the therapist, of teaching the patient about intimacy, love, or sex. Some of these therapists have had poor psychotherapy training and do not understand transference. Others respond to pressure from the patient.

Grandiosity is a common characteristic of those who become in-volved with patients. The therapist's character problems can support feelings of omnipotence and grandiosity that make rescue efforts seem appropriate. A therapist who is anxious about setting limits or who can-not tolerate a patient's rage and frustration can be seduced by the need to placate a patient who is perceived as provocative or demanding. The therapist may try to placate the patient by acceding to sexual demands. This is rarely placating for long, and the patient can then feel aban-doned and enraged. Some compartmentalize what they know in one context and do not apply it to another.

> A female doctor who was a fellow in addiction medicine was persuaded
> by a patient on the verge of discharge from an inpatient facility that he
> had nowhere to go, that it was a critical time for him, and that the doctor
> could save him from a disastrous crisis; she took him into her home tem-
> porarily, not realizing that he was drinking and also using drugs. They
> became sexually involved, and only later, when she had difficulty extri-
> cating herself from the relationship and getting him to leave, did she rec-
> ognize his addiction.

Although relationships with physicians other than psychotherapists tend to be less prolonged, they can be intense, and the situations are provocative in different ways. The obstetrician-gynecologist is con-fronted by the patient's sexuality and during training must work to desexualize and depersonalize the encounters with sexual information and with the genitals. Other physicians deal with nakedness and expo-sure of sexual material as well. For some, the physical examination is exciting or provocative and provides a context in which the usual ex-amination can become sexualized.

Who Are the Patients?

Just as there is no one therapist profile, there is no one patient profile. It is important to recognize that there are many factors, including the spe-cific nature of the patient's psychopathology, that increase his or her vulnerability. Often the patient's "pathology" has been blamed for the sexual involvement. But although the patient may be sexually provoca-tive, the therapist has the responsibility to take appropriate action, and blaming the patient's provocations or demands is another way of shifting responsibility to the patient. It suggests that the therapist is unable to control his or her responses to the patient's "pathologically" motivated provocations. The diagnosis of borderline or histrionic personality disorder, although clinically accurate in some cases, does not relieve the therapist of responsibility, nor does it describe the particular dynamics of the interaction.

This shift of responsibility to the patient's pathology is similar to other forms of sexual abuse in which the victim is blamed. For example, rape victims have been blamed for inciting rape by wearing "provocative" clothing or being in the wrong place (Notman and Nadelson 1976), and victims of sexual harassment are accused of stimulating and enjoying their encounters. Patients who have been sexually involved with therapists are subjected to the same suspicions and accusations.

In addition, the issue of consent can be confusing. It has been argued that sex between patient and therapist is an act between "consenting adults." This claim does not take into account the power of the transference in limiting the patient's freedom to choose and in enhancing the therapist's appeal. There have been some rare situations when a relationship has developed between a former patient and her doctor that have involved true consent. Some transference can persist; nevertheless, the patient has choice, depending on the nature of the treatment relationship, its duration, etc. Marriage does not change the dynamics of the original doctor-patient relationship, and if the marriage does not last, the former patient may feel exploited.

Attitudes of the Profession

Many therapists have encountered patients who have had a sexual relationship with a previous therapist or doctor. Despite knowledge of these liaisons in the professional community, there has been considerable reluctance to acknowledge that these relationships really occurred and were not the patient's fantasy and that they were damaging to patients. There has been denial of the possible truth of the accusations and reluctance to believe direct or indirect supportive evidence. In some instances, ethics committees have believed that they did not have sufficient data to reach a conclusion about the occurrence of the relationship; sometimes in these cases evidence is discounted or a patient's obvious psychopathology is used to discredit her story. Even when patient accounts have not been challenged, there has been reluctance to proceed with investigations or to take other action.

Sometimes the offenders are prominent in the community, and the sexual relationship appears to be inconsistent with others' experiences of them. Ignorance, lack of clarity about appropriate channels for reporting, the desire to protect the confidentiality of the patient, and the reputation of the offending therapist all play a part in colleagues' reluctance to acknowledge these violations.

Patients who have had sexual relationships with therapists describe the persuasive effects of the transferential authority of the therapist, and they often are not in a position to leave the relationship. The therapist may contribute to this by forbidding the patient to talk about it and even isolating her from peers and family (Wohlberg 1993). Former patients have expressed resentment about what they see as mutual protection within the profession.

In the past, the profession tended to rely on the power of supervision and psychotherapy to change the behavior of offending therapists. More recent experience has indicated that this has not been effective for many offenders—particularly those with serious character pathology, who may not be entirely honest with a supervisor or therapist. In addition, the power of psychotherapy to effect a change in these offenders is limited. For some, long-term psychotherapy is effective, but for others, disciplinary actions may be the only solution. Both are sometimes necessary.

Acknowledging that a colleague has had a sexual relationship with a patient can threaten the collegial relationship and demand painful confrontations. To some extent, denial and rationalization serve to increase the distance between oneself and the offending colleague and to make the possibility of one's own vulnerability to such involvement more remote. This distancing also protects against painful feelings of anger, loss, disappointment, and disillusionment at a colleague's betrayal of a patient, the profession, and oneself (Notman 1993).

The Dynamics of Boundary Violations

Therapeutic boundaries are not always precise or clear. There are gray areas, such as how one determines what is appropriate touching with children, the elderly, or those who are medically ill. A patient can also misinterpret a therapist's behavior as seductive or sexual. A therapist may fear that he or she will be viewed as cold and unresponsive, perhaps repeating in the transference the patient's experience with cold, rejecting parents. Such a therapist may put an arm around a patient or make other gestures that he or she believes are warm and caring but that can be experienced by the patient as seductive and sexual. This confusion is more often a problem for an inexperienced or poorly trained therapist. These problems occur in nonpsychiatric or non-therapist interactions with patients as well. The touch meant to be reassuring can be experienced as provocative. However, many of these relationships are grossly violating.

Understanding the power inequalities in the therapeutic relationship is essential to understanding boundary violations. If the therapist is male and the patient is female, the dynamic repeats the societal power differential. In the transference the patient responds to the person in authority—the therapist—with conscious and unconscious feelings brought to the therapeutic relationship from past experience with authority figures. Past adaptations, such as needing to please or gaining love by acquiescence or seductive behavior, can be brought into the relationship as if they were responses to the actual person of the therapist.

The patient's expectation that the therapist can heal accentuates the power that he or she attributes to the therapist. The power and authority vested in the therapist leave the patient vulnerable to influence and exploitation, which can often be—but is not necessarily—sexual. This vulnerability to boundary violations by the therapist can also exist in other spheres of the patient's life, including decisions about employment, finances, and relationships.

In all of these encounters there is a loss of therapeutic neutrality and a distortion of clinical judgment. Responding to the needs or demands of a patient with action, rescue attempts, or restitutive maneuvers without adequate understanding is a common therapeutic problem. When the response involves crossing therapeutic boundaries and engaging in sexual relations, it becomes unethical as well as clinically inappropriate. In situations in which the therapist is a woman and the patient is a man, the initial dynamic is often rescue wishes on the part of the therapist.

The inequality in power between men and women in society contributes to the fact that most sexual violations occur between male therapists and female patients (Vasquez 1991). The abusing therapist may not even be consciously aware of the power of his or her position and the impact of even seemingly innocent words or actions. For example, the therapist who persistently compliments a patient on her appearance may believe that the communication is a genuine statement of admiration or a means of showing support to an insecure woman. The patient, however, may hear the compliment as seductive and may feel that it violates the boundaries of the relationship. It also may represent a sexual interest that the doctor himself is not aware of.

The therapist who approaches a former patient may rationalize this behavior as acceptable because the treatment is over. To do so is to disregard the power of the transference—which exists even after termination—and the coercion that is implicit when there has been, and still is, an inequality of power. The therapist's narcissism or neediness may not allow him or her to perceive the ongoing transference-countertransference aspects of this interaction.

Even after therapy has ended, the transference is never entirely resolved. Thus, sexual contact after termination is influenced by some of the same transference issues, similar to parental or other authority and the enhanced appeal of the person with power. A relationship between a therapist and a former patient is not just any relationship. Therefore, sexual contact after therapy has ended has also been considered a boundary violation (Gabbard and Pope 1989; Vasquez 1991). There is much debate about whether time limits after termination can or should be imposed beyond which a sexual relationship is ethically permissible (Appelbaum and Jorgenson 1991).

Some women sexualize many of their relationships with men. Consciously or unconsciously, they negotiate their relationships with flirtation or seductiveness. In the therapeutic relationship, these feelings and behaviors need to be understood, verbalized, and worked with, not acted on. This is a complex dynamic and is more common between female patients and male therapists.

It is also important to recognize that in many relationships, the power or authority of a man is sexually appealing to a woman. Many women are attracted to a fatherly man or a man with strength. This attraction derives from normal developmental processes. However, in a therapeutic relationship this attraction is not based on knowing the therapist as a real person, and the transferential aspect of the relationship becomes distorting.

When boundary violations occur, patients often internalize blame and do not acknowledge or report transgressions by a therapist. The patient usually feels guilty and devalued and may also be embarrassed about being exposed as "sick," "weak," or "responsible." Furthermore, the patient may have concerns about the consequences of the sexual relationship, including rejection by a spouse. Guilt and shame may lead to unconscious denial and interfere with the ability to express anger.

Female patients who have been sexually abused by therapists often have a history of prior sexual abuse by a "powerful" man such as a teacher or father. It appears that, as with many forms of victimization, previous abuse does increase vulnerability to later abuse (Herman 1992).

The concept of traumatic sexualization has been used to explain the process of internalizing sexualized behavior as a mode of relating when there has been early sexual abuse (Finkelhor and Browne 1985). In this situation, the patient generally has had a long early history of abuse and so "learns" that the way to relate is by what we would interpret as sexualized behavior. He or she usually considers this behavior "normal," and it becomes a standard way of interacting. Thus, seductive behavior and sexual acting out may be part of the individual's behavioral repertoire, making her or him more vulnerable to subsequent victimization.

Therapists can also be victimized by unjust accusations; these appear to be relatively rare (Schoener 1990), although they may increase as more attention is focused on this issue. Probably more frequent, as we implied above, are situations in which a patient misinterprets the remarks or behavior of a therapist. For example, some patients feel that taking a sexual history is equivalent to intrusively crossing a boundary, even though it is generally accepted that sexual problems are an important and often neglected part of the psychiatric history and possibly a source of a patient's distress. In assessing the patient's complaint, it is important to ascertain the context in which the information is obtained and the therapist's manner—for example, whether the interest appears to be appropriate to the history or appears to be out of context, persistent, or overly detailed.

Treatment Issues: Subsequent Therapy

The Therapeutic Alliance

The subsequent therapist inherits to some extent the transference problems of the former therapist. The critical issue in any subsequent therapy with a patient who has had a sexual relationship with a therapist is building trust and a therapeutic alliance. Trust in another therapist is difficult to establish, and for some it may not be possible. Some patients never return to therapy. A therapist who is too detached, intellectual, or remote, or one who seems overinvolved or too invested in his or her own agenda, can be experienced negatively by the patient. An empathic response to the patient, an acknowledgment of the distress that has been caused, and the capacity to express these feelings to the patient are essential to optimal treatment. The therapist cannot be the judge of the veracity of the patient's report, although some authors have suggested that the more unusual the story, the more likely it is to be true (Apfel and Simon 1985b).

The therapist must be flexible and consistent and must maintain appropriate boundaries. An oversolicitous or overindulgent attitude, such as the failure to end hours on time or to charge a fee, can be experienced by the patient as another boundary violation.

For many patients who have had sexual relations with a therapist, maintaining control over the therapy is extremely important, and sometimes they may need to maneuver in ways that can seem unnecessary to others but are extremely important for them to feel safe. Some patients may need to dismiss one or more subsequent therapists before being able to work with someone. Attitudes and behaviors that in other circumstances would be possible to work through can in this situation be enough to put the patient off. The therapist may have difficulty allowing the patient to maintain enough control—especially if control takes the form of manipulative and demanding behavior—and at the same time appreciate, respond to, and validate the patient's feelings.

The therapist must also be aware that the patient may be repeating patterns from early experience, possibly with an abusing parent, and must remain empathic when faced with provocations to be punitive, judgmental, or seductive. On the other hand, if the patient perceives the therapist as helpless and despairing, he or she may identify with that affect and feel that it is not possible to recover. A patient's experience of sexual abuse by a therapist is usually profoundly damaging to self-esteem, and the patient may be labile and insecure. The therapist who is anxious, who avoids the patient's affect, or who defensively seems to protect a colleague risks alienating the patient. One does not have to take a position on the details of the events to recognize, appreciate, and respond empathetically to a patient's distress.

In many ways, therapy subsequent to this form of abuse is like any other therapy, although there are some aspects that warrant emphasis. Many of the symptoms of posttraumatic stress disorder (PTSD) are present, and the therapy employs some techniques used to treat PTSD patients. Repetition is common. The patient may need to tell the story many times, and the therapist must be willing to hear it repeated and to deal with the associated affect. Victims of this kind of sexual abuse talk about the importance of having the therapist validate the "whole" story; it needs to be heard in its entirety and affirmed by the new therapist (Gabbard and Gabbard 1989).

As indicated earlier, some patients who have been sexually abused by a therapist are so traumatized that they are unable to seek subsequent therapy, or it may take many years before they will risk going into therapy again. The anger and disillusionment they experience can be so overwhelming that it takes several attempts before they can express and tolerate the intense affect. They may also reaffirm control by dismissing a therapist who is found wanting.

Treatment Issues Existing Before Abuse

An important and sometimes neglected aspect of this therapy involves recognizing that the issues that originally brought the patient into therapy may never have been resolved. Exploring this possibility requires, as in any therapy, a thorough understanding of the patient's history. However, it is important to balance the need to understand the patient's history with the urgent need to give attention to the distress and to respond to the abuse. Some patients complain that the therapist's efforts to connect the abuse with his or her history are either "pathologizing" a real-life trauma or using a stereotyped psychiatric approach rather than dealing with the hurt and destruction caused by the abuse. This may seem to them to be insensitive and rigid, and it can provoke anger or rejection of the therapist. In addition, the intense negative affect that the new therapist can feel toward the prior therapist, the desire to avoid revictimizing the patient, and the therapist's difficulty in tolerating the patient's anger may lead the therapist to avoid this important exploration.

After working through the issues of trust, the aftermath of the sexual abuse, and the patient's earlier concerns, patient and therapist must also understand the sexual encounter in terms of the patient's life and experiences, including any prior psychopathology. To ignore the way in which the sexual experience fits in with the patient's earlier concerns is to deny the patient the opportunity to heal. It also leaves the patient with the potential stigma of the abuse.

For many patients, the subsequent therapy can eventually resolve both the abuse experience and the original presenting problems. Some patients, however, remain profoundly involved with the posttraumatic aspects of the abuse and may organize their lives around it. These patients may be particularly difficult to treat; the major goal of treatment is to help the patient move beyond the abuse, and these patients may be unable to do so without a major therapeutic effort.

Transference and Countertransference

One of the most important tools of psychodynamic psychotherapy is the transference. As we indicated earlier, the transference provides an important source of insight into the patient's past experiences and also into responses to people in current life. Psychodynamic issues from past experience that may have contributed to the patient's complying with the therapist's sexual demands are reflected in the transference. These can be the patient's need to please, relationships to people in authority, vulnerability, or other factors. The emergence of erotic feelings with a subsequent therapist can cause the patient to experience anxiety, shame, and guilt. The patient may feel out of control and fearful that the new therapist will also be exploitative (Pope and Gabbard 1989). The countertransference responses of the subsequent therapist are also important to recognize. Erotic countertransference feelings may occur in response to a patient's erotic transference feelings. The therapist may also feel curious and have a voyeuristic interest in the patient's story.

The therapist must be aware of and be able to deal with these feelings or they are likely to interfere with the therapy. Consultation and supervision to discuss these issues are recommended whenever feasible.

Countertransference can also be manifested in the new therapist's anger at the abusing therapist. This can be so dominant that the therapist cannot treat the patient unless action is taken, such as reporting the previous sexual relationship. The intensity of the affect aroused can interfere with the therapist's objectivity and the ability to be an empathic listener. This anger can dominate the therapist's reactions to such an extent that the patient's agenda can be lost. Any ambivalence the patient feels can be hard to express if the new therapist takes a strong or rigid position. The therapist must be sensitive to the patient's wishes and degree of readiness to pursue action.

The subsequent therapist who becomes so preoccupied with retribution or with punishing the offending therapist that the patient's autonomy and control are sacrificed can actually revictimize the patient. As indicated earlier, communicating a sense of helplessness, impotence, or fear can also impede empowerment of the patient. Some tolerance and endurance are necessary to help the patient come to his or her own decision, when the decision is within the patient's control and not mandated by law.

Boundaries

Maintaining appropriate boundaries in the subsequent therapy is particularly important. A therapist who feels sympathetic to the patient and wants to be especially nice to the person who has suffered may be tempted to prolong hours or offer extra support in the form of special treatment. This can be more problematic than helpful, because it can be perceived as a loosening of boundaries and can challenge the patient's confidence in the therapist's ability to maintain boundaries. A failure to charge a fee can be experienced as another boundary violation. To maintain appropriate boundaries and at the same time be flexible and empathic is a clinical challenge.

Some patients will be provocative to the subsequent therapist or invite punishment or critical judgments. The therapist needs to recognize that these are most likely repetitions from earlier experience and avoid leaving a therapeutic position for a judgmental one.

Positive Feelings Toward the Abuser

Anger is not the patient's only feeling; other feelings, including positive ones toward the abusing therapist, may also need to be recognized (Gabbard and Pope 1989). The patient may be reluctant to discuss the previous sexual relationship or to report it because of these positive feelings, which can persist despite the anger. The patient's acknowledgment of ambivalence involves the recognition that the offending therapist may also have provided attention and caring and that the therapy may even have been helpful in some ways. This is not unlike the positive feelings the incest victim can have toward the perpetrator. Acknowledging these positive feelings in the subsequent therapy also supports the patient's self-esteem because it can provide validation and understanding of why he or she remained in the relationship. Sometimes the abusing therapist is charismatic, and the sexual relationship can seem special, at least for a time. A more "ordinary" subsequent therapist can then appear dull and less powerful.

Sometimes the patient who has been sexually involved with a therapist has had the fantasy of being the therapist's favorite patient, or perhaps the only one with whom there was a sexual relationship. Acknowledgment that this is not so can bring a real sense of loss and disappointment. This realization and the feelings that follow sometimes enable the patient to break off the relationship or to report it.

Reporting and Advocacy

Reporting sexual abuse by therapists is mandated in some states. This requirement can have a major impact on the therapy. Some have recommended that the therapist forewarn the patient about the limits of confidentiality and the mandated responsibility to report, if that is the law (Gabbard and Gabbard 1989). The patient can then decide whether to withhold identifying information. It is essential, however, that mandatory reporting not take the place of therapeutic responsibility to work out the meaning and effects of reporting; this responsibility exists regardless of whether reporting is mandated.

Reporting represents a potential violation of confidentiality. For the therapist this can be inconsistent with continuing in the therapeutic role. If possible, advocacy and therapy should be separated. The patient can be referred to another therapist, either for consultation—with the goal of having the consultant report, advocate, or give testimony in court—or for continuing the therapy. The same kind of dilemma exists in relation to the therapist being the patient's advocate.

The problems of combining advocacy and therapy are not limited to issues of confidentiality. The therapist's advocate can inhibit the patient's freedom to explore all the feelings related to the abuse and to talk freely. Negative transference feelings can interfere with advocacy. The patient needs to feel free to bring any feelings and be sure they will not influence the therapist's position. The therapist's success or failure in relation to a court appearance has countertransference effects as well. Court appearances or legal involvements are not usually consistent with ongoing psychotherapy.

For the therapist, mandatory reporting may provide relief from the burden of decision making, especially regarding confidentiality. It may also be a relief for a patient who is hesitant to report. On the other hand, mandatory reporting can also prevent the patient from working through his or her own feelings and exercising autonomous judgment.

An important countertransference problem connected with the question of reporting is the therapist's possible identification with the abusing therapist. This can be expressed as skepticism and even subtle blame of the patient. It can also take the form of being overprotective of the patient or overly concerned with the potential negative consequences of reporting or taking action. The therapist's usual orientation toward understanding rather than action can also contribute to anxiety about stepping out of this role.

Conclusion

It is clear that sexual encounters with therapists are profoundly damaging experiences for patients and that they have long-term consequences. In some ways these experiences are similar to other traumas. However, particularly in the effects of subsequent therapy, these experiences are unique because the violation occurred within the therapy. The patient needs to resolve the initial reasons for seeking therapy as well as work through the effects of the experience. The intense and complex transference and countertransference issues may be continued in the subsequent therapy, and they may provide some insight for the subsequent therapist who is sensitive to his or her own responses. Many of the clinical dilemmas can be addressed by obtaining consultation or supervision.

As more attention is paid to sexual violations in therapy and more clinical data accumulate, it will be possible to understand more about the motivation and dynamics of therapists who engage in this behavior. Several strategies are indicated. Education and the clarification of boundary issues and limits are important; these efforts must avoid a reductionist approach that ignores the complexity of the issues. Attention to transference and countertransference issues and the availability of nonpunitive consultation and supervision to help a therapist deal with these problems at an early point are important. Also important is a recognition of the limits of training and psychotherapy for therapists who are repeat offenders, as well as greater knowledge of and sensitivity to character traits that may contribute to such behavior. Grandiosity, omnipotent fantasies, and charismatic qualities can accompany therapeutic gifts, but they also appear to characterize some of the therapists who become sexually involved with patients.

References

Apfel RJ, Simon B: Patient-therapist sexual contact. I: psychodynamic perspectives on the causes and results. Psychother Psychosom 43:57–62, 1985a

Apfel RJ, Simon B: Patient-therapist sexual contact. II: problems of subsequent therapy. Psychother Psychosom 43:63–68, 1985b

Appelbaum PS, Jorgenson L: Psychotherapist-patient sexual contact after termination of treatment: an analysis and a proposal. Am J Psychiatry 148:1466–1473, 1991

Finkelhor D, Browne A: The traumatic impact of child sexual abuse: a conceptualization. Am J Orthopsychiatry 55:530–541, 1985

Gabbard GO, Gabbard K: The female psychoanalyst in the movies. J Am Psychoanal Assoc 37:1031–1049, 1989

Gabbard G, Pope K: Sexual intimacies after termination: clinical, ethical, and legal aspects, in Sexual Exploitation in Professional Relationships. Edited by Gabbard GO. Washington, DC, American Psychiatric Press, 1989, pp 115–128

Herman J: Trauma and Recovery. New York, Basic Books, 1992

Notman MT: Countertransference reactions to a patient's sexual encounter with a previous therapist, in Beyond Transference. Edited by Gold JH, Nemiah JC. Washington, DC, American Psychiatric Press, 1993, pp 159–172

Notman MT, Nadelson CC: The rape victim: psychodynamic considerations. Am J Psychiatry 133:408–413, 1976

Olarte SW: Characteristics of therapists who become involved in sexual boundary violations. Psychiatric Annals 21:657–660, 1991

Pope K, Bouhoutsos J: Sexual Intimacy Between Therapists and Patients. New York, Praeger, 1986

Pope KS, Gabbard GO: Individual psychotherapy for victims of therapist-patient sexual intimacy, in Sexual Exploitation in Professional Relationships. Edited by Gabbard GO. Washington, DC, American Psychiatric Press, 1989, pp 89–100

Schoener G: Frequent mistakes made when working with victims of sexual misconduct by professionals. The Minnesota Psychologist, 1990, pp 5–6

Simon RI: Psychological injury caused by boundary violation precursors to therapist-patient sex. Psychiatric Annals 21:614–619, 1991

Twemlow SW, Gabbard GO: The lovesick therapist, in Sexual Exploitation in Professional Relationships. Edited by Gabbard GO. Washington, DC, American Psychiatric Press, 1989, pp 71–88

Vasquez MJ: Sexual intimacies with clients after termination: should a prohibition be explicit? Ethics and Behavior 1:45–61, 1991

Wohlberg J: Boundary violations. Workshop presentation at the annual meeting of the American Psychiatric Association, San Francisco, CA, May 1993

INDEX

*Page numbers printed in **boldface** type refer to tables or figures.*